All proceeds from the sales of *TERMINAL* support the
LESLIE'S WEEK Vacations Away from Cancer.

To Nancy,

Thank You for helping me through all my rough times
I couldn't have done it without you!!
You are a true inspiration to all. Just like
my DeAnna ♡. Keep up the fight never give
up! I am so glad God brought us together from
DeAnna ♡ Love you like a sister. I so enjoyed our
weekend together- Twinzie!! Call me or text me anytime!

Love You

Y.S.

TERMINAL

STRAIGHT-FORWARD BLUNT

LESLIE'S WEEK STAGE 4 BREAST CANCER
COLLABORATORS CLUB of
"NONFICTION WORDS THAT READ LIKE FICTION"

43 AUTHORS

17 STAGE 4 BREAST
CANCER WOMEN

12 HUSBANDS

13 FAMILY MEMBERS

SANDRA GUNN

ISBN-13: 9781076382061

Editorial Supervision by Sandra Gunn

Book Cover and Illustrations by *Anonymous Artistes* in support of LESLIE'S WEEK
Book Design by Danielle Joyner

Printed by Kindle Direct Publishing in the United States of America

First Printing Edition 2019

Self-Published by:

LESLIE'S WEEK

www.lesliesweek.org

THE LESLIE'S WEEK STAGE 4 BREAST CANCER COLLABORATORS CLUB
DEDICATE THIS BOOK TO

All Stage 4 Breast Cancer Women Across the Planet in Every
City - Town - Village - Parish - Hamlet - Hut - Shelter

We dedicate this to you who live TERMINALLY on the edge of the breast
cancer community; raise your voices and come into the light.

"There are no shortcuts to anyplace worth going."

TABLE OF CONTENTS

TERMINAL

PREFACE

THIS BOOK IS about Metastatic Breast Cancer. It is a family disease. It impacts every person in the family community. There is no cure. It is terminal.

Breast cancer affects women of every age, ethnicity, and socio-economic class. In fact, 1 in 8 women will develop breast cancer in her lifetime and over 30% of them will have Metastatic Breast Cancer. Hearing the words, "You have breast cancer", is one of the most significant events in a patient's life. It can trigger huge emotions, such as shock, grief, anger, and despair.

Most women hear the words, "You have breast cancer", from an interventional radiologist, breast surgeon, or their primary care provider following a breast biopsy. Some are told over the phone, while others have waited many anxious hours to be told in-person at a follow-up appointment. It is a moment for which no one is ever fully prepared.

This is not a technical, medical, disease descriptive book. We do not define anything other than the Stage 4 Metastatic Breast Cancer Journey from those who are taking it and have taken it. Their heartfelt words are profound and moving. It defines a husband's love beyond any experience known to those who are not afflicted with Stage 4 MBC. These men endure emotional pain on unimaginable levels, in silence, to protect their children, while cherishing their wives.

A woman with Stage 4 Breast Cancer loses much of what society says defines her femininity. She loses her breasts to Mastectomies. She loses her hair to Chemotherapy. Her skin burns and peels with Radiation. She looks in the mirror and no longer recognizes the image reflected back to her.

The husband watches as his wife's breast cancer metastasizes to her lungs, brain, bones or liver. She is no longer the glue that holds the family together. No longer in her realm of responsibilities are household duties, shopping, laundry, lunches for the children, driving them to school and after-school activities. The family is losing income as she is unable to work and may now struggle to pay the mortgage and other necessities. He too misses work to drive her to appointments with surgeons and oncologists, for chemotherapy and radiation treatments. He watches in silence.

Children are traumatized by experiencing the slow decline of their mother, the first woman they fell in love with. They have no frame of reference, no language with which to use in their expression of their fears and anxieties. They may become isolated and withdrawn. Their grades and social skills may decline and they become the *watchers* of their mother's pain and slow death. They too are silent.

This is a book written by the LESLIE'S WEEK STAGE 4 BREAST CANCER BOOK COLLABORATORS CLUB, whose "nonfiction words that read like fiction" will leave you breathless. Our more than 43 COLLABORATORS are not writers; they are Partners in Breakthrough. This book is written to break the silence and give a voice to the women and their families affected by Stage 4 METASTATIC BREAST CANCER. This is a family disease.

And, this is written for You.

I dare you to take this journey with us. You will never be the same.

Sandra Gunn
Founder and CEO

INTRODUCTION: LAUREN HUFFMASTER
I am Breakthrough

WORDS ARE SOCIETY'S most powerful way of framing the issues of our time. For thousands of years, philosophers have discussed how language affects perception. The words we use, shape our filter around an issue; yet in the age of people-first language and politically correct speech, there remain many blind spots where we continue to utilize labels that feed into outdated and inaccurate perceptions. Living in an era of medical and technological breakthrough, we must often embrace new labels for our thoughts to grow and change with the times.

Individuals living with cancer are one of the groups that have been held back by old labels. Currently, it is acceptable to call anyone impacted by cancer a *cancer patient*, or *cancer survivor*. Why have these labels been allowed to identify more than 17 million individuals living with cancer in America? We do not name someone with diabetes a *diabetes patient*. People-first language teaches us that a person is more important than a disability/disease. So why do we continue to allow cancer to be more important than the individuals it effects and use our speech to determine that a disease can define a person's identity?

To gather perspective on these labels let us look at their origins. From the 1940s until the 1980s, there were very few, if any, effective treatments for those with a cancer diagnosis. The term *cancer patient* was an accurate descriptive in that time. There were few cancer survivors. A person with a cancer diagnosis was without choice except to submit oneself to the guidance of a doctor. Little to no information was available, and therefore, anyone with a diagnosis of cancer could be correctly labeled a *cancer patient* because many of these patients would not experience life after cancer. In the 1980s, with the rise of technology, there came effective imaging and screening for cancer. For the first time, the death rate of cancer patients began to decline, and a scientist spoke for the first time of *cancer survivors.* The new term caught on because there was new hope for cancer patients, the hope of survival.

Neither of these terms accurately describe a person impacted by cancer today. By definition, *patient* is an individual who submits his/herself or is acted upon by a physician. Though this may have been accurate 20 years ago, it no longer is an accurate description of cancer treatment. Presently, within hours or days of receiving the news of a diagnosis of cancer, one is given treatment choices and is urged to make significant treatment decisions, immediately. I have personally known multiple individuals who were given the choice of which treatment to receive first chemotherapy or surgery. The implications of such a decision are significant, yet as a newly diagnosed patient, such a choice is often decided by when it would be convenient to be sick for 3 to 6 months. In the moments after diagnosis, most of us have no idea what type of questions to ask to help make such choices, and usually, no one is there to help guide us. Furthermore, studies show that for the newly diagnosed, the fear that fills the mind minimizes decision-making skills and limits one's ability to process information around such stressful decisions.

But this example shows how those impacted by cancer design their own treatment choices, even within minutes of a new diagnosis. Once an individual is diagnosed with cancer and moves beyond the initial shock, they will soon learn of a plethora of treatment paths available. By talking with other individuals impacted by cancer or researching treatment plans from physicians around the world, an individual impacted by cancer can become empowered with a variety of available treatment paths. Cancer treatment is a dynamic process, a two-way discussion, and there is no expectation of quiet submission.

Let's look at the term *cancer survivor* and its implications for a person impacted by cancer today. Until a cure/vaccine is the typical treatment for every individual impacted by cancer, there is a large population of people who question the label *cancer survivor.* Today, many cancer treatments only postpone cancer's impact on lives. In some situations, treatments themselves may kill the current threat of cancer in a body. However, it will go on to create cancer over the following 5 to 15 years. Other treatments may only push cancer back to a level where it can no longer be detected but then again discovered at a later date. Today's label of *cancer survivor* is misleading and inaccurate. Those impacted by cancer long for the day when every individual who receives a cancer treatment will be called a *true survivor,* and not simply living for a five year benchmark, but living long, full lives without fear of cancer's return.

We are living in an era different than those that created the labels of *cancer patient* and *cancer survivor*. Today there is a whisper of a cure. Every individual impacted by cancer sits on the edge of their seat, thinking, *"The next big breakthrough could save my life, and so I will combine knowledge and wisdom and push myself so that I may be standing when that breakthrough comes for me."* It is a new era for the community impacted by cancer, and it is time for a new identifying term.

In this age of breakthrough, attention is focused on fundraising and the large research entities racing to glory. In the excitement, though, we have forgotten that for every medical breakthrough during these last twenty years, there have been thousands of engaged patients who chose to participate in clinical trials, risking their lives for a cure. In this breakthrough era, those affected by cancer continue to die from treatments. In fact, they must. Someone must provide the data. Someone must be resolute enough to present themselves to try what has not been tried before. Physicians and researchers cannot change treatment norms without participants in their studies. Individuals affected by cancer must risk their lives every day in pursuit of a breakthrough, in pursuit of a cure.

Yet, when and where have we ever celebrated their courage? On a t-shirt? On a hat? With a color? As a young adult living with Stage 4 Breast Cancer, I must say I have never felt more alone than in the month of October when stores suddenly turn pink. There is no face attached to the sales. There is one marketing ploy after another, and it feels completely disconnected from the people it says *pink* represents. There is no mention of the individuals impacted by cancer. There is no mention of me.

How, as a society, do we recognize the courage and sacrifice of hundreds of thousands of individuals living among us with cancer? While they wait for a cure, those impacted by cancer offer up their lives in pursuit of a medical breakthrough. It is their strength that overcomes the odds to reveal what is possible. Those impacted by cancer are the driving force of medical change. They are the breakthrough. So instead of labeling them as *patient* or *survivor*, it is time to acknowledge their place in finding the solution to cancer. Progress cannot occur without them.

"I am not an unengaged patient. I am reading the research. I am designing my own treatment plan. I am changing the statistics. I am living longer. I am not yet a "true survivor," but I am a Partner in Breakthrough."

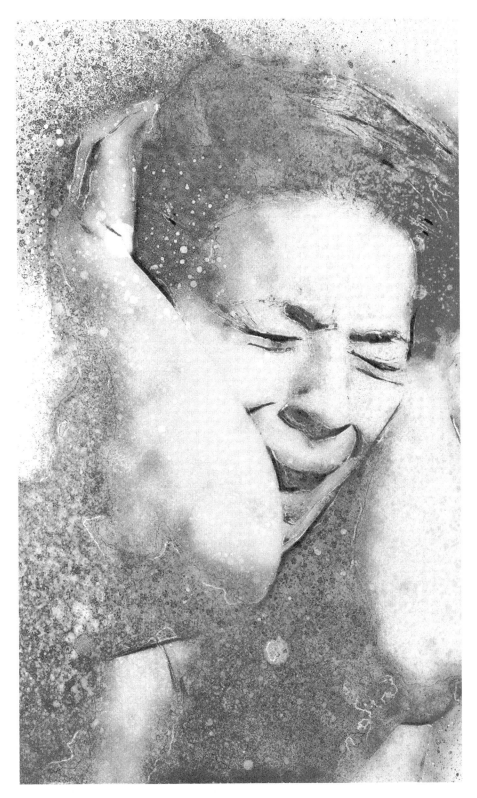

01. THE WOMEN
"I HAVE WHAT?"

I WAS SITTING AT my desk. The phone rang. I answered it. "Hello, this is Sandra."
The voice replied, "Mrs. Gunn, I am sorry to tell you that you have breast cancer."
I replied, "I have WHAT?"

The radiologist was kind, but in a hurry, as he had other breast cancer calls to make. We discontinued our call. I was speechless. There is no evidence of breast cancer in my family. I exercised daily at the gym, ate whole foods, never fast foods. I'm healthy, have never been on prescriptions except for the occasional antibiotic, and have been a happy human for the greater part of my life. I gathered myself.

My GP gave me the name of a surgeon she highly recommended and I made an appointment to see Dr. Lorraine Tafra. My husband, the GunnMan, and I were sitting in a small comfortable area when she entered and introduced herself. She asked, "How do you feel about your breasts?" I thought that was hilarious and responded, "They came in handy when I was nursing our two sons." We sort of laughed and then she went on to discuss the process that was about to introduce me to the Breast Cancer world.

The class I attended prior to surgery was called the 'Gear Up Workshop'. I did not have Stage 4 Breast Cancer. I had Stage 1. There were fifteen of us in the class and I was the only Stage 1. It was on that day that I was introduced to the word *METASTATIC*, I had never heard it before. They were Metastatic; I was not. When I heard the stories of their Stage 4 Metastatic Breast Cancer Journey, those women changed my life forever. They began my quest on that day for Stage 4 Metastatic Breast Cancer women and their families.

This book is about Stage 4 Metastatic Breast Cancer women and their journeys. They and their husbands will tell their stories in their words. You will be profoundly moved. These stories are intended to educate and inspire patients, future patients, their loved ones, and the next generation of health care professionals.

Come, take this passionate journey with me into the world of Stage 4 Metastatic Breast Cancer women and their families. They will captivate you with their candor, innocence, and clarity. You will never be the same after you read their "nonfiction words that read like fiction".

ERICIA LEONARD Hearing those words...

I was at work and I actually had an appointment to see the surgeon the next day. My phone rings and I hear those dreaded words, "You have Breast Cancer!"

My very first thought was OMG it's my daughter's birthday today how am I going to pick up the cake? How will I be able to maintain? I called my husband and we both left work and met at a park. I couldn't go home because my kids were there. He just held me and we cried.

I was so worried about him because his dad died of cancer and I felt like I did something wrong and now he has to deal with this again. The next day at my appointment the surgeon talked with us so long he sent his staff home to continue talking and went from A-Z. He was awesome.

My second time was worse. I had to go to the ER because I forgot how to talk and read[1]. Honestly, I thought I was having a stroke. When the ER doctor came in with three nurses I knew it was bad. I just kept saying out loud "not again, not again." It was all I could do to breathe. There again, my first thoughts were of Erik. How strong he had been since the beginning and how I failed him and our kids. How I could have, should have done more.

TINA ARGO Hearing those words...

I was floored when I was told I had breast cancer. My mind couldn't take another one.

You see, I know cancer way too well. I had cardiac amyloidosis[2] and multiple myeloma[3] and fought them for a long time to achieve remission. Now along comes breast cancer, ugh. I laid my head down. My OBGYN told my mom and I we can do

---

[1] These symptoms would occur with Brain Metastasis

[2] Cardiac amyloidosis is a disease in which clumps of proteins called amyloids build up in the heart. Over time, these proteins replace normal tissue, leading to heart failure.

[3] Multiple myelomas is a cancer of plasma cells

this! I said, "I am not ready to do this again."

All of my family comes in and gives me support telling me I can do this. What they don't get is, it is hard to fight especially with chemo that ravaged my body. Yes, I am whining and I have a right to. As I prepare my mind and talk to God about me fighting this I stand tall and proceed onward with it.

The first chemo treatment put me in the hospital with dehydration. It was a nightmare. Our small-town communities don't know how to deal with all this cancer stuff, but I got through it. Then next chemo I stayed close to the treatment center and ended up in the hospital with dehydration again.

The Doctor asks, "When did you eat last?"

I said, "It's been seven days." He tells me he will make sure I eat in the hospital.

After pondering and getting advice from a very trusted individual, I decided that chemo wasn't for me. I have been told I still have amyloids inside of me, which are dormant. It makes things super sensitive for my body so I can't do chemo or I will not make it through the next one. I prayed to God and asked him for a sign. He gave it to me. My decision is to let God take the whole lead now and he will decide my fate with how I will endure through this journey.

DENISE HAYES Hearing those words...

I was scheduled for a mammogram and ultrasound. The tech told me an ultrasound would only be needed if the mammogram seemed abnormal. The mammogram was complete. She said let's do this ultrasound. Once the ultrasound was complete, the tech informed me that the radiologist would like to talk with me.

They NEVER talk to you!

My heart sank. The look on his face said it all as he sat in front of me. He held my two hands and told me he was very concerned with what he saw. His words knocked the breath out of me!

It was my grandson's birthday, June 17th. How was I supposed to function? I surely was not going to ruin his party!

I was scheduled with the surgeon 2 days later. Waiting for the results took forever. Their confirmation of breast cancer was not as shocking as being told I was metastatic from the get-go after I had been told I was Stage 3^4. I was pregnant.

MELISSA ZIEMIAN Hearing those words...

At 36, while breastfeeding my first child, I felt a lump in my left breast. I was assured by my doctor that it was from breastfeeding since I was young, healthy and lacking a family history of breast cancer. I was told when I was 40 I could get a mammogram. My second daughter was born eight months later. The lump was still there and I was assured it was nothing to worry about.

I received a negative report from an ultrasound screening event that I attended. I was the *healthiest* person I knew, running half marathons and eating clean. Five months after the ultrasound my youngest wouldn't sleep more than 20 minutes. One night she refused to nurse on my left breast. That was when I knew something was really wrong and I truly believe she was telling me this.

The next morning, I made an appointment and was diagnosed four days later over the phone. There simply aren't words that can describe the roller coaster of emotions that followed. I was 39 then and facing Stage 2 Breast Cancer, which was re-diagnosed to Stage 3C after surgery revealed more disease than initially expected. This news crushed me more than the initial diagnosis, which itself was devastating. I felt guilty for not listening to my body sooner and for trusting my doctor at the

---

[4]Breast Cancer Stages: BreastCancer.org

Stage 0 is used to describe non-invasive breast cancers, such as DCIS (ductal carcinoma in situ). In stage 0, there is no evidence of cancer cells or non-cancerous abnormal cells breaking out of the part of the breast in which they started or getting through to or invading neighboring normal tissue.

Stage I describes invasive breast cancer (cancer cells are breaking through to or invading normal surrounding breast tissue) Stage I is divided into subcategories known as IA and IB. Stage IA describes invasive breast cancer in which: the tumor measures up to 2 centimeters (cm) and the cancer has not spread outside the breast; no lymph nodes are involved. Stage IB describes invasive breast cancer in which: there is no tumor in the breast; instead, small groups of cancer cells — larger than 0.2 millimeters (mm) but not larger than 2 mm are found in the lymph nodes or there is a tumor in the breast that is no larger than 2 cm, and there are small groups of cancer cells, larger than 0.2 mm but not larger than 2 mm in the lymph nodes.

Stage II. The cancer has grown, spread, or both. IIA means the tumor in the breast is still small if there's one at all. There may be no cancer in the lymph nodes, or it may have spread to as many as three. A stage IIB breast tumor is bigger -- it may be the size of a walnut or as big as a lime. It may or may not be in any lymph nodes.

Stage III. The cancer has not spread to bones or organs, but it's considered advanced, and it's harder to fight. IIIA means the cancer has been found in up to nine of the lymph nodes that form a chain from the underarm to the collarbone. Or it has spread to or enlarged the lymph nodes deep in the breast. In some cases, there is a large tumor in the breast, but other times there's no tumor. IIIB means the tumor has grown into the chest wall or skin around the breast, even if it hasn't spread to the lymph nodes. IIIC means cancer has been found in 10 or more lymph nodes or has spread above or below the collarbone. It's also IIIC if fewer lymph nodes outside the breast are affected but those inside it are enlarged or cancerous.

Stage IV. Breast cancer cells have spread far away from the breast and lymph nodes right around it. The most common sites are the bones, lungs, liver, and brain. This stage is described as "Metastatic," meaning it has spread beyond the region of the body where it was first found.

time. Maybe I was relieved to hear it was okay, although deep down I was skeptical. Wasting time on guilt was not helpful and I quickly realized that everything does happen for a reason.

Surrounded by love, support, and purpose, I quickly entered fight mode. I didn't realize that hearing the words *"you have breast cancer"* could be more devastating until two years later when I heard the words *"your cancer has returned and metastasized."* My first thought was, I am going to leave my girls without a mother and my husband a widower. This was not supposed to happen, not to me. But it has and I will remain in fight mode for the rest of the life that I am so blessed to have. I will never stop fighting, never stop praying, and never lose hope.[5]

TERESA TEAFORD Hearing those words...

I left work early that day with not a worry in the world. Alone and confident this appointment was pointless. Cancer didn't run in my family. If it was cancer I wouldn't have felt breast pain and I'm only 35 years old. I was called back into my OBGYN office as soon as I walked in. Before I even had my butt in the chair the doctor spoke the words, "I guess you know you have cancer."

I was confused, angry, and scared to death as I walked out of his office alone.

I had no one to lean on so I held myself high and walked to my car where I finally allowed myself to break down. I sat in the parking lot for over an hour trying to figure out *"why me?"* Then I had to break this news to my family, my husband, and three kids. I'm not sure the kids really understood, but as I cried they cried. All I could do was reassure them I was going to be okay. Even though I wasn't confident in my own words.

I was uneducated about cancer — that to me meant a death sentence. Chemotherapy was my only hope at survival. It was the road I had to take if I wasn't ready to leave this earth. This is where my story begins.[6]

---

[5] Melissa died on Christmas Day, December 25, 2018

[6] Teresa's daughter Teya left high school to become her mother's caretaker. In Teya's words, "I have been taking care of my mother since the first time she was diagnosed with breast cancer. I've been to every chemo, every scan, every checkup, everything! I actually ended up becoming homebound (online classes) my last two years of high school because I became moms primary caregiver. I have always pushed my mom to do things that are out of her comfort zone. I make her try new things and go to new places. I try to get her to live her best life because I am aware I could lose her any day now."

I knew my life was not complete. There was a calling, something set apart for me as I was set apart for it.

The years that led up to my initial diagnosis of cancer I had daily reminders of 11/11. Every day on a clock, or a sign, or a book I would see 11/11. I thought that November 11 would one day hold the biggest joy of my life. So, year after year I would show up to work on November 11 declaring that something amazing was going to happen! This was MY day, something HAD to happen! And nothing, nothing, nothing.

Then in 2015, I met with a gynecologist who sent me in for a mammogram. On 11/11/15 I was told I had breast cancer. I will never forget the doctor handing me a doctor's note saying, "From 11/11/15 to 11/11/16 Lauren Huffmaster will not be available to take care of anyone but herself." Though I fought it for a month or so, she was right, my survival depended on my ability to rest.

My first diagnosis I processed as a trial. Who doesn't have trials? I have a wonderful life, an amazing husband and family. If I must be tested, let it be in my physical nature. No problem. I held onto my God's faithfulness and inability to fail and kept walking. No problem 11/11/15 to 11/11/16. I can do this.

At that time, I knew no one in my own town and was served by the kindness of strangers for a year. I received support and love that poured in from all over the country. I experienced love because of my situation. I experienced God's faithfulness, and I remained faithful to Him as I moved through the trial. I had deep communication with God through my darkest moments and I never doubted. I loved others whom I met in cancer circles and I was open about my struggles. I walked through the trial pulling from the faith that I had built in my spirit throughout my life.

For two years I pursued the list of treatments that were given to me on the initial night of my diagnosis: chemo, mastectomy, radiation, reconstruction, reconstruction adjustments, and oophorectomy[7]. In December of 2017, I met with a surgeon about my impending oophorectomy, the last item on my list. I went to have a PET/CT, as is expected before any surgery. Then on 12/21/17 my doctor called me with tears dripping from her voice and heard that I have Metastatic Breast Cancer. The cancer spread through my spine and my pelvis, with multiple tumors and lesions.

For all that had altered my life under the first diagnosis, nothing compares to this

---

[7] An oophorectomy is a surgical procedure to remove one or both of a woman's ovaries. The surgery is usually performed to prevent or treat certain conditions, such as ovarian cancer or endometriosis.

news. There is no "from this moment until that moment you will have cancer." This is a diagnosis for the entirety of life. This is a diagnosis without a cure. A diagnosis with no hope at the end of a tough battle. This is a diagnosis that demolishes my understanding of a trial. This is completely unexpected; a possibility that never crossed my mind.

All of my life, the prayer of my heart has been, "Here I am, take me, use me." Over the past two years, I have met so many cancer survivors. I have laughed and cried with them. I have shared their pain, fears, anxiety, hopes. They are family. Even before I meet a newly diagnosed cancer patient, I know them. I love them and hurt for them. We are bound together.

My First Descents[8] family, a group of survivors, describe us as a tribe. I have been called to this tribe. There are a large number of young adult survivors in our country who are hurting, hopeless, desperate, and alone. I have been initiated into this group through cancer. I love these people because of cancer. I will serve these people because of cancer. Cancer, for me, is not a valley tucked between two mountaintop experiences. Cancer is the calling of abundant life. It is my broken state through which God can best display His love. It is my weakness through which God's power can be perfected. It is the one thing I can boast in because I believe His greatest work in my life will come through it.

I know a thousand voices have raised prayers for my healing since I announced my diagnosis but it is not the prayer of my heart that I may be healed. I simply pray that I may rest in God's plan. There is a plan. It is not what I was expecting God's calling to look like, but there is a calling. I feel overwhelmed by the idea that God would set apart a tribe of hurting, dying people, that I may be love to them. It is both the worst and greatest realization of my life. Though I do not want cancer in my life, I embrace it as my earthly sacrifice. In the walking out of this sacrifice, I find the purpose I have longed for my entire life. So, when you pray, pray not only for me but for young cancer survivors around the world. Pray that I may be a voice of peace, a voice of love.

AMANDA HOLBROOK Hearing those words...

When I was told I had breast cancer I felt like I was outside of my body looking at someone else's life. It's one of "those things" you hear about all the time but it is

---

[8]First Descents is a nonprofit that offers adventure-based group therapy to adult cancer survivors.

happening to other people. You think it would never happen to you. The first couple days didn't feel real. I was getting a lot of flowers and gifts from friends and it was because this horrible thing was happening to me. I mean, who doesn't like gifts? It was a very confusing feeling, torn between gifts and breast cancer diagnosis. It took two to three days and then the tears came.

I remember the day the sadness finally hit me. Of course, it was a dismal day all around. It was dark and raining all day long. I spent the day sobbing in bed under my covers. My wonderful partner kept the kids busy and brought me food and drinks, though I didn't eat or drink much that day. That was the day I started mourning for my life as I had known it because many things were about to change.

DEANNA RAYMOND Hearing those words...

The day my life was changed forever!

March 5, 2015: I was sitting in my doctor's office room patiently waiting for my results from my biopsy after waiting for them for less than a week. I was thinking to myself, *"I just turned 29 this has to be nothing."* My one and half-year-old son was getting into everything in the room and I'm trying to keep him quiet and entertained while I nervously wait.

All these thoughts are going through my head like, *"Why am I waiting so long? Wasn't my appointment a half hour ago? Does this mean something bad or maybe it's a good thing? Should I have brought someone with me today? This waiting is killing me! The unknown is killing me, but yet I'm only 29 I'm sure I'm fine."* I keep telling myself that it's going to be OK, take deep breaths, you're fine!

My son is getting agitated, he wants my attention and I can't seem to get in the playful mood so I give him my phone to entertain him. Finally, the doctor walks in with his nurse right behind him. My thoughts were this isn't good! He sits down and I'm starting to feel a little sick to my stomach.

My palms are sweaty and those words come out of his mouth, "I'm sorry, you have breast cancer!"

I immediately pick up my son and wrap him in my arms. I am numb. I have no emotions, no feelings, nothing, just nothing. He goes on to say, "We have you set up for two appointments; one is to see a breast surgeon and the other is for an oncologist."

Still numb, he asks if I'm OK? I nod and reply, "Yes."

I am still not sure what just happened. It didn't sink in until I made my first phone call to my mother and then I broke down. I couldn't even get the words out of my mouth. I was crying so hard still not knowing really anything other than I have breast cancer. I finally get those four words out and she starts crying. We are both crying and I tell her I have to let her go. "I can't drive like this with the baby in the back seat. I need to calm down and drive."

My second call was to my fiancé. At the time I don't think he believed me, he just kept saying, "No! This can't be right, no." He just watched his uncle die of lung cancer two years ago, this was all too familiar and this was a road he didn't want to go back down. I finally get myself together and start the truck and head home. He left work and met me there, the rest of the night was spent drinking a few beers and talking with my mom and going over the results I had taken home with me. That's the day I will never forget. That's the day I started this crazy journey. It is the day my life changed forever!

JEANETTE RHILE Hearing those words...

First, some background:

My initial diagnosis was in June 2010. I survived this diagnosis with hope in my heart.

In early 2017 I was having discomfort in my chest and shoulders so I went to my plastic surgeon in March 2017. He said my pain was not caused by my reconstruction implants and sent me to my oncologist. She said it isn't the cancer, but let's do a CT scan anyway. I had not been granted a scan since my initial Stage 3 diagnosis in 2010[9].

When I went back to see her to get the results, I was alone because she had said it wasn't cancer. I wasn't worried and, besides, they didn't tell me to bring anyone with me. She marched into the room and bluntly announced, "its back in your liver and bones."

I was stunned! I had done everything to fight this, how is it possible that it is back already!? I had to drive myself home, the longest fifteen minute drive of my life. I stopped at my husband's work to collapse and sob in his arms.

---

[9] Patients with early-stage breast cancer are considered cured after treatment. Although they will continue to get annual mammograms, no other imaging (CT, PET, MRI) is routinely done unless there are physical symptoms of recurrence.

I was diagnosed with Breast Cancer in November of 2015. I saw an indent on my left breast. What ran through my head was my bra caused it. I asked family members and friends in October, who are RN's, and they told me to watch it and call my doctor if I saw any change. I thought it would go away in time.

At that point in my life, I changed jobs and was in my second week of training. It was November of 2015. When I noticed that my indent was longer, I freaked! That is when I went to see Dr. C., I was late on my yearly checkup by a few years, life got in the way of making that appointment. The moment Dr. C came into the door he knew I was scared. And believe me, I was! He knows I am strong! But during my exam, he had a face that I could sense something was wrong with me! He said I needed to go to the hospital and get a mammogram immediately. They showed me the mammogram results, I saw the difference immediately but they didn't tell me what it was.

Luckily my mother in law and father in law were with me. We got to the hospital and my heart sank that I needed this. After the mammogram, I was told to wait for the results. I waited. It seemed like forever to me! They showed me the results with Dr. G. That is when they told me I needed a biopsy. They didn't wait another day, let alone another moment! And damn the biopsy hurt, lots of cussing and crying, but I knew I needed to do it. I started to pray asking this to be nothing. All I could think of was I couldn't handle another thing. I was married to my husband Scott for fifteen months when our family was hit with his unexpected loss in September of 2014.

I had an appointment with Dr. G the next day and that's when I found out with Ryan, my partner, that I had breast cancer. All I could think of is, *"I want it out. Take it out!"* That was the plan, I even saw a plastic surgeon for implants. I kept thinking of all the things I did wrong. Why didn't I take the time to get my yearly checkup? Why didn't I put myself first? When did I get this?

A few days before the surgery I had a bone biopsy on my L3. I was having pain there since September 2015. My eight hour surgery was scheduled for January 2016. I was prepped and waiting to go in with my mom by my side. Things didn't go as planned that morning. 5:00 AM was too early to call Dr. G. When I saw him thirty minutes before surgery I was going to ask him some questions but then I saw Dr. T behind him. Something isn't right! I knew it even with the happy juice. That was the moment I was told that the cancer had metastasized to my L3 and we weren't doing the BIG surgery. I was going to get a port put in and start chemo the next day. It didn't go as planned.

I started my chemo treatment and that put me in the hospital. The bathroom was my best friend. The treatments kept me in bed and ultimately made me sicker than I ever thought I could be in my life.

My priority was always the kids first and then myself. But at times I had to put ME first. It was painful to see my kids go through this cancer and see me the way that they did. They knew Mom was really sick and I wasn't getting better. All I thought about was I have to get through this for them! They've been through enough with losing their dad and some of their family on his side and now me having breast cancer!

I am fighting hard! I have my moments when I didn't want to fight anymore, I wanted it to end but I look at them and I know that is not an option. It never will be an option. Throughout the months of chemotherapy, radiation, and now maintenance chemotherapy I've found out that my life will never be the same. But that's okay with me because I am here! I am kicking ass! I am going to continue to kick ass head on and be that strong, stubborn bitch that I am.

I am coming up on year three since my cancer diagnosis. Metastatic Breast Cancer life expectancy is three years. Scary to think of if you ask me. Have I done everything that I wanted to do in life? No! Hell no! My kids are only eight. I'm thirty-four years old. But I will continue to live my life to the fullest with my kids happiness first and foremost. I have another round of chemo tomorrow, number forty-six to be exact. My cancer has been maintained!

That is what we want as Metathrivers. We want to maintain. We are never curable! Ultimately Stage 4 breast cancer is going to kill me.

SHELBY QUINLEY Hearing those words...

Late October 2003, I noticed a lump in my left breast about the size of a small marble. I went to the doctor, Dr. K. who gave me a *feeling test* and told me that we would watch it. He told me with me being only twenty-six years old that it was likely not something to be concerned about.

After talking to family, I made the decision to go back to the doctor and have the lump removed. He removed the lump with a procedure in his office. That was a nightmare and scary as hell. On November 13, 2003, he called me to tell me I had breast cancer. He said, "Don't worry, it is slow growing."

All of this resulted in me having a double mastectomy in a nine hour surgery, by a different doctor, Dr. B. The surgery was followed by six months of heavy chemotherapy and five years of medication. I was told I was more than likely not going to be able to have kids due to all of the medication. This was another blow to me, as I had always wanted kids. Anyway, life went on.

SARAH LEVINSON Hearing those words...

I noticed over the summer that I had a small pink rash on my left breast. It wasn't getting worse and sometimes seemed to be going away, so it definitely didn't trigger me to think about breast cancer. Then in October, I was looking through Facebook posts and a friend of mine posted something unusual. She reposted a graphic with the symptoms of inflammatory breast cancer (IBC).[10] That was the first time I had ever heard that you don't need a lump to have breast cancer!

A Google search later I found out that inflammatory breast cancer was a rare form of breast cancer that accounts for one to five percent of all breast cancers. Surely, I couldn't have self-diagnosed something so rare! I tried to push the thought of cancer out of my mind. Then, a few weeks later after going to bed, I noticed my left arm felt funny. I had been cleaning the garage that day, but I thought it was odd that only my left arm was bothering me, especially since I was right handed. I couldn't sleep so I Googled "arm pain and breast rash." The rash was back and getting a little worse now. I pulled up some more info on inflammatory breast cancer. What I read wasn't good in that it is only diagnosed atSstage 3 or 4 and that only fifty percent of patients survive five years! Completely freaked out, the next day I was able to see a nurse practitioner at the midwifery group that I had been going to for the past seven years. They had helped me to birth the last two of my three children. I asked her if it could be inflammatory breast cancer and she replied that "No, it's too rare." But she would send me for a mammogram anyway to find out what's going on. Having just turned thirty-nine, I had never had a mammogram before, even though at my last GYN exam I had asked for a baseline mammogram at thirty-eight. I was told it was better to wait until I was forty[11].

Having not had a mammogram before I didn't realize how unusual it was that I got a follow-up ultrasound immediately afterward or how the radiologist doesn't usually meet with patients. When I spoke with the radiologist, again I asked if it could be inflammatory breast cancer and again, she replied "No, it's too rare", but

---

[10] Symptoms of Inflammatory Breast Cancer (IBC): Redness of the breast, swelling of the breast, warmth, orange-peel appearance, other skin changes, swelling of lymph nodes, flattening or inversion of the nipple, aching or burning.

[11] Approximately 67% of women age 40 and older get a screening mammogram every one or two years.

she said that the next step would be to get a biopsy to find out what was going on.

The next day my husband and I met with a breast surgeon and I was lucky enough to get an immediate in-office biopsy. Again, I asked her if it could be inflammatory breast cancer, and again I heard, "No, it's too rare", but we would get the pathology back the next week and figure out what's going on. Finally, a week later, the day before Thanksgiving, we were back at the breast surgeon's office. She had us come in as the last appointment of the day and we waited in the exam room for what seemed like forever.

My husband looked visibly upset, as a healthcare provider, he knew that waiting so long wasn't a good sign. Finally, she came in with a serious gaze and said that I had breast cancer. In a moment, my world had changed completely. It took me a moment to come out of shock. I thought about the diagnosis at that moment and resigned myself to that fact that many people get diagnosed with early-stage breast cancer and recover.

"So okay," I asked, "what kind of breast cancer is it?" The next thing I heard was, "It's inflammatory breast cancer." That's when I felt the sudden, grave devastation and replied with a pleading, "But I thought you said it was too rare."

SANDRA GUNN Last words...

After reading this I am as stunned now as I was then when those courageous Stage 4 breast cancer women in my "Gear Up" class told me their greatest fear was, *"What will become of my children after I am gone?"* Never thinking of themselves but always thinking of those they leave behind. Unselfish, suffering in Silence, and always mindful of those they love. They leave a glow when they die. I've seen it.

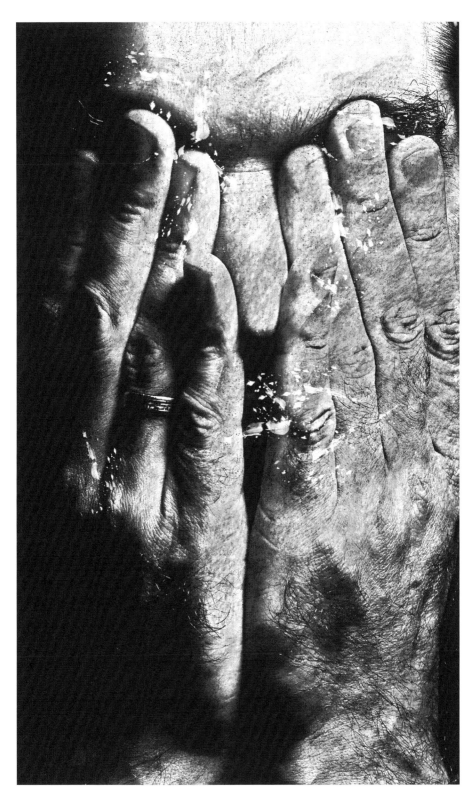

02. THE HUSBANDS

"You said what?"

WHO ARE THESE MEN whose love and loyalty to their family prevails over all temptations they face in their lives? Who are these men whose steadfast sense of responsibility moves them to endure with their wives her pain, depression, and declining health? Who are these men who watch everything that defines a woman removed from the women they love?

Think of this, their wife and the mother of their children is diagnosed with Breast Cancer. It grows to Stage 4 and metastasizes to her lungs, brain, bones or liver. She is no longer the glue that holds the family together. She is gradually unable to continue household duties, shopping, laundry, clothes and lunches for their children, driving kids to school and after-school activities, perhaps holding down that second job that helps pay the mortgage and other necessities. They pick up the slack in all she did for the family.

They drive her to her appointments with surgeons, oncologists, chemo and radiation treatments. They sit with her in her room after surgery and wait. They are vigilant as they watch over her. They hold her when she falls. They help her with her wounds and medications. They keep a face of love for her to see in her direst moments. They laugh when inside they are crying, for every day they feel like they are losing her.

Their company decides they have missed too much work and they are laid off. Their savings and other investments are diminished or depleted in their efforts to keep their wife alive. Their family financials become Toxic. They find two jobs to keep the bills paid. They spend time consoling their frightened children who look up to them as hero dads.

They live intimately with Stage 4 Breast Cancer, but mostly in silence. They are isolated and forgotten. They live in the background. Their wives are where the attention is focused.

CLIFTON HUFFMASTER Hearing those words...

Certainly, I'll never forget the day my wife told me she had Stage 4 breast cancer, and that the Stage 3 breast cancer that we thought we had eliminated only six months earlier, had already spread to her spine. For one thing, she woke me up with the news, so that for the next month or so, I always had the feeling that maybe it was a bad dream from which I would soon wake. Nor will I ever forget the day, the same day, actually, that I sat in the oncologist's office and asked her point-blank: "About how much longer do you think my wife will live?"

Of course, what I really said was, "What is my wife's prognosis?", in a sorry attempt to sound smarter than I am. Naturally, the oncologist gave me the least definite answer possible. She literally said, "Well, if we didn't do anything at all she would still live for one more year. But, on the meds we're going to put her on, she could live like five to ten years or more." Wow, I thought, that's one hell of a spread. So, you're telling me that she is going to live somewhere between one to ten years, or more?

But, truthfully, none of these things that "I'll never forget", I kind of hate that phrase, but it is just so true, is really what I wanted to talk about. The *'but'* at the start of this paragraph was supposed to be a major contradiction, a huge turning-point thing. Because, the thing that I remember most, (*a better way of saying that I'll never forget? Sort of like, the thing I'll never forget the most?*) is the time that I realized that it makes no difference how much longer my wife lives if I spend the entire time in a state of mourning. If the years I get to spend with her are filled with grief and sadness at the prospect of what is coming in the future, they will be wasted years.

What I choose to remember from that horrible time in our lives, is that it doesn't have to stay horrible. I can decide to be joyful. I can pick peace. I can live the remainder of my time with my wife, no matter how long it is, with exuberance. I'll grieve when the time comes; I'm not going to mourn while she is here with me. Not only would it be stupid to grieve while she is here, I literally can't do it. I cannot live in mourning for the next ten years. I just can't.

That is not to say, of course, that every day is perfect and that I never get sad. I do. It sucks. Besides, on the other hand, (*another big 'but,' I guess*) it is also good for us to grieve together. I think that sometimes, she needs to see me cry. She needs to know that she is going to be sorely missed. She has to know that I'm mourning too. So here I am, I think, walking the tightrope as it were. Attempting to choose joy, trying to embrace the time I have left with my wife with gratitude and happiness, but at the same time, never fearing to let the tears fall, not only for my sake (*there is healing in tears*) but for hers too.

BRIAN QUINLEY Hearing those words...

We were at the ballpark for my son's baseball game. My wife took the *phone call* and was sitting down crying in the parking lot. It was such a private moment which was exposed to everyone at the ballpark.

My kids started crying (*they didn't know why*) and all I could think of was that I needed to get everyone home. We had driven separately and I made sure one of the kids rode home with her so she could focus on that and then completely break down after she made it to the house.

She had Stage 4 metastatic breast cancer. ALL of life changed.

RICHARD WARD Hearing those words...

I'll never forget the day that we first heard the words, *Stage 4.* It was the most terrifying day of my life. I kept praying that it was a mistake. Everything around me slowed down and all I could think about was there had to be a cure. This can't happen to us. There has to be something I can do to fix this.

This was over a year ago but those things still run through my head today!

THOMAS NEWMAN JR. Hearing those words...

When I heard Breast Cancer I thought, *"we can get through this."* When I heard it's through her bones like *"fine shot."* That was a bad day!

CURTIS ARGO Hearing those words...

My wife called me after she left the doctor's office and the words she said were, "I have it again babe." I will never forget them, they are etched in my soul. I was so mad and angry! I mean why her again? She has already been through all of it!!!!!!

When she was put on the maintenance drug for her Multiple Myeloma we were told she could get secondary cancer, but never did I dream she would. I would sit and think, "How will she make it through this again, the sickness, the hair and all the agony of trying to get well." This made me so sad that I knew what was coming up ahead for us, either I would lose her, meaning die, or she would go way down with all the chemo. Well, the ER visits started as soon as the chemo hit her body. She couldn't eat and had tried but the chemo dehydrated her enough that she couldn't even stand. I had to help her do everything. When the doctor came in and saw her he kept her there till she could eat again.

I can't comprehend how anyone can leave their wife going through this ordeal? I wasn't backing down and I would be her support through all she had to do. I knew the worst part would be her losing her hair cause it made her sad the last time she did. This time she made it fun. She dyed it hot pink before surgery then as chemo started we shaved it all off. I saw her tears falling and I held her and told her, "You can lose whatever you have to but I will always love you."

In our mind, she is the center of our lives and we will value all of the time we have, we take one day at a time, Things are slow now and that is okay with us.

Life is what matters now and we live by that.

MICHAEL BANK Laurin Bank is leaving me.
September 24, 1988 – October 21, 2018

To: The World and My Husband
From: Laurin Long Bank

Well, this will be a Polka Dot Wednesday that will go down in the history books for this journey! The third time of going to try to get one more triple dose chemotherapy was not the trick. It actually led me to one of the hardest conversations I have had with my oncologist! A conversation I knew was possible all along. A conversation I was hoping would not come until 5 years from now but that is not the case!

I met with my oncologist today to be told the fluid in my belly was most definitely cancer. And that my body cannot handle any more chemotherapy and more than likely the cancer is in my bone marrow due to the fact blood work has gotten worse each week instead of better. The cancer is spreading like wildfire and the strongest possible dose of chemotherapy they can give me did not work. I am now to the point that chemotherapy is no longer an option. Due to that and the bone marrow issues, this also shuts the door for any clinical trials!

I am at peace with the fact that since I was diagnosed with breast cancer on September 11, 2014, that I have treated this the most aggressively as possible and researched the best possible doctors. When I was diagnosed last year on August 2, 2017, with Stage 4, I have taken the path of the most aggressive possibilities and researched the best doctors. I have been blessed beyond measure with an amazing medical team from day one! I am grateful that I have an oncologist that was so honest and open with me today about my condition and he cared enough about me to still allow me to have the quality of life I have left so I can go make memories with my husband and travel!

This is one of the hardest days in this journey for me and I know I am still processing. I have shared from day one that this is a part of the journey and I plan to share all the adventures and updates I can and until I can't.

My husband and I plan to make the best of everyday and travel as much as possible so if you have an extra room let me know I may end up in your city! Our number one goal has always been to have fun!!! We plan to make LOTS of memories!

The plan to go forward is Friday. I will get drained one last time and I will also have my meeting with hospice that afternoon as I was talking with the social worker today to get that setup! Tuesday I will have a procedure to get a port for my abdominal fluid so I can drain the fluid from home! I am moving to home healthcare, moving forward unless something falls out of their realm of coverage! Less time at the hospital so I have more time with my loved ones and able to travel again!

I just want to keep things as normal as possible as long as possible! Making the best of each day and making memories are my wishes going forward!!!

I can't thank everyone for all the love and support I have received and I just want to say THANK YOU!!!!! Mike and I have been so blessed with amazing support and love from so many! We appreciate it so much!

We are still processing the information received today so if you do contact us just know it may be a delayed response as this is A LOT to

process and a huge transition for our very new family unit to go through!!
Like Mike said at least we are in this together!

Will update when I can! Again, if you contact, just know my response
may be delayed.
So much love,
Polka Dot Queen

*P.S. Always remember riding topless = happiness ;) such a beautiful night to ride in
the convertible with my love!*

JOSHUA LEVINSON Hearing those words...

Nearly three years after a stone-faced doctor gave Sarah a terrifying diagnosis — we
sat again, tortured, waiting for results. Sarah's oncologist walked in the door. I quickly
read his face for a preverbal diagnosis. Without uttering a word, he smiled and raised
both thumbs up. "The cleanest PET scan I've seen in a year...no evidence
of anything."

For the second time in three years, Sarah has *no evidence of disease.*

"And what happens next?" Sarah asked.

"We don't know," he said.

Nearly one year ago – just one year after chemo, mastectomy, radiation and *no
evidence of disease.* Sarah was diagnosed with a re-occurrence of breast cancer. This
time it had spread to her lymph node above her clavicle and a PET scan found
inoperable cancer in a lymph node between her heart and ribs, Stage 4 Breast
Cancer. This is bad because the lymph node is a door to the entire lymphatic system.
The node is a filter for a (*lymphatic*) system of fluid (*not blood*) whose job it is to get rid
of waste in the body. It is assumed that cancer cells could be floating anywhere in
her body.

Sarah and I have gone through a nightmarish roller-coaster ride of daily despair,
resolution, despair again, and possibly some resolution. In the weeks following her
diagnosis of a Stage 4 breast cancer recurrence, her doctors finally agreed on a
treatment plan. With this recurrence, Sarah and her doctors decided to hit cancer
hard and treat it with everything possible. Sarah completed a course of A/C (*the red
devil*), a red chemotherapy infusion. She endured twice daily radiation for four weeks
and developed nasty burns, couldn't eat or swallow without pain and developed
secondary infections requiring hospitalization. Finally, Sarah officially finished eleven

weeks of her last chemo (*Taxol*), Herceptin and Pejeta targeted antibodies (*non-chemo drugs*) and continue infusions every three weeks. PET scans will continue every three months.

Although the prospect of infusions sounds terrible, we are relieved that there is hope. In the strange new normal that is our lives, Sarah and I are looking forward to spending every bit of time with friends, family, our children, and each other.

RYAN CASSIDY Feeling Thankful

Breast Cancer has taught me several things I would never have learned in life. The past two years have been enlightening, emotional, aggravating, exciting and exhausting. Cancer has a tendency to take and give. It has taken from me the chance to share once in a lifetime experiences with my best friend/partner and her munchkins due to the condition she has been dealt. But far greater than that, it has gifted me the opportunity to look at my best friend every day like I had never seen her before. Because every day is a gift. Holidays come only a few times a year, but for me, it is every day. Today is Danielle's thirty-third birthday. And while she may be stubborn, bullheaded and sarcastic, she is also loving, giving, beautiful and smart. I hope everyone gets something from this because every day is not given to us. Every day is a gift. What will you choose to do with it?

RYAN AYARS Hearing Those Words...

It started off as chronic back pain. Keeli has had back pain all of our marriage, so this wasn't a surprise or really even a big deal. We'll have the doctor prescribe some painkillers and see what we could do to fix any of the ailing vertebras.

We had recently discovered that Keeli had Stage 1 Breast Cancer. The plan was to have a lumpectomy, move on, and become a *survivor*. The Dr. had requested a scan, due to the recent pain she was feeling in her back, so we went to the cancer center to go over the results. We sensed that something wasn't right, because the staff was gearing us up for some bad results.

The doctor came in and communicated that the pain was due to tumors that had spread from her breast to her spine. "This is what we call Stage 4 cancer," he said.

"So, what does that mean?" we said.

"It means that this is what will most likely kill you sooner than when you would have died. We will need to go over a treatment plan to begin shortly," he said.

The rest of the conversation was a mix of cancer buzzwords and theoretical timelines, all of which I can't say I understood. They moved us to a private room, while the nurses came in and asked the needed questions. The next couple of hours were probably the worst of my life filled with fear, anxiety, sadness, confusion, etc. I wouldn't put this kind of thing on my worst enemy.

The idea that kept going through my head was, *"Your wife is going to die and there is nothing you can do about it but wait for the inevitable."* It's a truly helpless position for a caregiver. However, my God-given duty is to be the rock for my family and that is what I'll do.

Fast forward to a year later, we found that there is another lump. However, nothing more is showing up in the scans, so Keeli will need to have back surgery, or *'mud jacking'* as she calls it. The tumors will be attacked individually with radiation treatment. Here we are, the two same people that almost crumbled, when first hearing the Stage 4 diagnosis, now we can take any diagnosis they throw at us. We are stronger than ever.

SHAWN RAYMOND Bad news today...

Unfortunately, we got bad news yesterday! Deanna had a CT scan done and chemotherapy in the office yesterday. We waited on the results because she has been in so much pain in her stomach! We found out the liver tumor that was only 1.1 inches on the 2nd of November is now 4.8 inches so it's growing fast. It's also triple negative. We hoped it might have mutated and been another cancer that would be easier to treat but it's not, so now we have to change our course of treatments.

MICHAEL ZIEMIAN

Tears streaming from her eyes...
December 20, 2018

Unfortunately, Melissa is even worse today. She can't talk, can't remember what year it is...really struggling. Still in LV Muellenberg hospital. Great care at the hospital but can't find the smoking gun. My mother in law and I were able to have a nice talk tonight so at least something positive happened. Sat with Melissa tonight and held her hand and prayed out loud. Tears streamed from her eyes so I know she's there...

I know she heard me...

December 24, 2018

Melissa means so much to so many that I felt it was the right time to let everyone know what's going on. Melissa was admitted to the hospital on Wednesday, December 19, and her physical health declined quickly over the course of the last 48 hours. Yesterday I made a decision to put Melissa in God's hands. She is now under the care of hospice inpatient at our local hospital in Bethlehem. Last night I got to spend the whole night with Melissa in her room alone. We prayed together and I spoke out loud about all the feelings I have for us and our two daughters. I know she heard me. This morning in concert with her Mom and two sisters we were able to bring Lily and Layla over to see their mother. It was an incredible visit. Melissa responded to their voices and their kisses. Melissa is comfortable. She is radiant and beautiful. Our families are having opportunities to see Melissa today. May God bless this angel and keep her in the comfort of His hands. We are taking things hour to hour and I will continue to keep you informed.

...she peacefully took her last breaths...

December 25, 2018

I am heartbroken to let you know that Melissa passed away earlier this evening. I got to sit with her in the dark listening to music holding her hand while she peacefully took her last breaths. Our daughters picked out this sweater for her to wear today at the hospital and Melissa's mom dressed her in it. Melissa is comfortable in heaven with three weiner dogs lapping her face off. Lily and Layla were asleep when I got home so I will be spending all my time tomorrow with them. I will provide any details about services at some point later. I hope everyone had a blessed Christmas...

SCOTT PETRONE Thoughts on Michael and all Husbands...

This pretty much sums up why I felt so strongly that the husbands, boyfriends, fiancées, and brothers needed an outlet and the opportunity to be among the other caregivers to our Stage 4 BC Women at our Vacations Away From Cancer at the DreamMore Resort. In time that will be expanded to mothers and fathers, aunts, uncles, and wives of Stage 4 MBC women. It has been a tough week or so for some of us. We lost a 2017 alum in Nina, multiple women had surgeries or agonizing chemo treatments, there were scans and the anxiety that goes with them. Right now, one of ours is in the darkest of places that we all have feared or experienced. Michael had to make the agonizing decision to leave Melissa's fate in the hands of God. Keep strong brother! I'm so impressed with how you have handled this last week. We are all part of your village, spread out across the country, but united in heart and mind. I am here for you, we are ALL here for you and for each other.

March 16, 2019

I can't emphasize enough how important it is that you all take care of yourselves! I'm talking mental, physical, spiritual…whatever! You all do amazing jobs taking care of your families, nobody will question that. But are you really taking care of yourselves? Think that five pounds, ten pounds, twenty-five pounds will go away? Think you are managing your stress effectively? Are you the best version of yourself?

I thought I was! Now, granted I am in a different situation that most of you having lost MaryAnn seventeen months ago, but that just means I have a new perspective. I was in a pretty deep depression, feeling like I couldn't even get out of my own way. I was feeling inadequate as a father, my girls were suffering from me being snippy, angry, and sad. I had no energy at all. I was eating garbage (*still am to a point, but getting better*), I was drinking too much. (*Not a drunk, but more than I should as the only responsible adult in the house.*) I was literally about to break. Fit me with my straight jacket and reserve my padded room!

Why do I tell you all this? Because I don't want you to be like me. The last eight months have been a much different story. I got the help I needed taking care of my girls so I can work and reduce my stress and anxiety. I got the mental health I needed by seeking out a professional to talk to. She has been great and I highly recommend seeking mental help if you need it. She has helped me realize that by doing my best, I will always be an adequate father. I also reconnected with God. I put my faith in him to guide me through this journey, even when I wanted to curse him for what has happened. I'm also in the final weeks of my conversion to become a Catholic — like my girls and MaryAnn. It has been an incredibly powerful journey for me to the point of tears a few times.

It doesn't matter if you are a widower like me, or a spouse/caregiver to your wife like most of you. You need to take care of yourself so you can be your best for your family! Are you going to have bad days? Yes. Are you doing to have bad weeks? Probably. I'm here to tell you that is okay. BUT, you still need to take some 'me time'. It's not selfish. It's not abandoning your family. It's life maintenance to make sure you are the best you that you can be!

I miss you all Stage 4 breast cancer husbands and the time we spent bonding at LESLIE'S WEEK. I pray for all of your families on a regular basis. Keep your heads up! You got this!

SANDRA GUNN Last words...

Who are these Men?

This is who they are!

Steadfast, loyal, loving, gentle, caretakers, caregivers, but sadly, they are mostly silent. Now their voices will be heard with LESLIE'S WEEK and this book they helped to write.

Heroes!

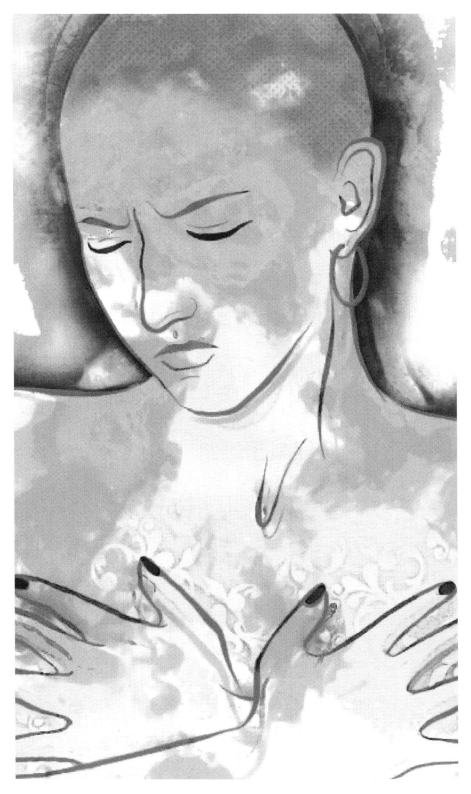

03. THE DIAGNOSIS
I am Metastatic

I WAS NOT METASTATIC.

I was Stage 1A when my first mastectomy occurred in April 2013. In the beginning, I didn't know what Stage 4 was. I only knew I was going to be okay. I was stunned when I attended the Breast Centers 'Gear Up Workshop' for all those being operated on that month. Among other things, it was to inform us of what to expect when we no longer had our breasts. Imagine that – *when we no longer had our breasts!*

There were fifteen of us around an oval conference table. The social worker asked that we introduce ourselves and describe our cancer. She picked me to start because I was sitting next to her. I just hate being first in that kind of situation. I am shy, even though no one who knows me would believe that.

I began with, "I am Sandra. I am being operated on April 4th and sure am glad it is not April 1st!" That comment broke the ice, then laughter, then seriousness. I told them it was a right breast mastectomy. We then proceeded around the table. One woman stuck out in my mind and remains there until this day. I could not see her well. She said, "I am expecting a bi-lateral mastectomy and am having implants using the TRAM flap procedure cutting tissue and muscle from the tummy."

I was fascinated and asked her how this is done? She

Transverse rectus abdominis muscle or TRAM flap

The illustration above depicts a free flap, in which the tissue is cut free from its original location and reattached in the chest area.

51

replied, "The skin, fat, blood vessels and at least one abdominal muscle are moved from the belly to the chest." I was stunned that anyone would consider what seemed to me to be a surgery on top of a surgery.

I said, "You are a brave woman!"

Her husband was sitting behind her and he said to me, "YES - SHE - IS!" He was proud and scared that he was losing her. He was exhibiting his love for her in front of all of us. I was moved to tears that I held back so as not to show emotion. Even as I write this my eyes fill with tears to honor his pride in her.

They were all Stage 4. I was Stage 1. I never met women like this. There was no self-pity, no arrogance, no ego, no false humility. There was a strong, silent determination that filled the room. They were each quietly sharing their disease with us. During breaks, I tried to meet each one and engage them in conversation. I asked each, "What is your biggest fear?", thinking they would say surgery, pain, disfigurement, death, experimental drugs, side effects. Not one of them said any of those. They all said, "What will become of my children when I leave? Who will love them as I do? Who will care for them, teach them, and guide them when I am gone?"

I had my surgery on April 4th, 2013. My family surrounded me in my room. I looked at my sons differently after that. I knew every moment counted for me from that moment on. I knew I could not afford one single distraction, not one single false relationship, not one single lost opportunity. It was there that I made up my mind to find a way to take their Stage 4 Breast Cancer cause to another level. You will never meet women like Stage 4 Breast Cancer women or men like their husbands. You cannot know them and remain unchanged.

Stage 4 Breast Cancer women lose everything that society defines us as women. The lose their breasts to surgical mastectomies. They lose their hair to chemotherapy infusions. They lose their skin tone to radiation treatments where their skin peels and finger and toenails fall off. They lose their nighttime sleep and their days to experimental drug side effects. They no longer recognize themselves when they look in the mirror. They stay positive, pray for a cure, look after their families with a love like no other. They keep their humor and their strength of conviction in their purpose. YES - THEY - ARE!

LAUREN HUFFMASTER
My Stage 4 cancer announcement happened like this...

After waiting six months after my treatments from Stage 3 breast cancer I felt my body was strong enough to proceed with a preventative oophorectomy. I scheduled it for after the holidays.

December 21st was the last day of school before Christmas break, so I ran in for my pre-op PET scan. I left the scan, picked my girls up from school and we came home to prepare for an end of school Christmas party with all of their friends. I expected twenty-five K-3rd graders to show up in two hours and we had cookies to make.

My three girls and I were wearing our matching Christmas aprons, busy with flour and sprinkles when my phone rang. It was the doctor. The Christmas music was cut off. Doctors don't call after a scan to give good news. She told me to come into the office, now, it couldn't wait. I looked around the room, red and gold and white lights everywhere, and the color just drained away.

I told her to just tell me, I didn't need to wait to be in an office with a bunch of strangers. The idea of her wanting me to have a breakdown in a place where everyone could see angered me. And so, she hesitated and told me the scans showed that my cancer has spread down my spine and into my pelvis and ribs.
I hung up the phone and went to wake my husband, who was sleeping before his shift. I was screaming tears. No part of me expected this. I just finished every treatment they told me to do! How is this possible? I screamed and cried in our dark bedroom until I noticed my neighbor in the door saying she was taking the children to her home. My husband was quickly making arrangements for my kids and the party, but I was lost in the darkness, unable to experience anything but grief.

My husband drove me to the oncologist's office, never letting go of my hand. The doctor really had nothing further to say. There were meds — "it could give me a couple years without progression. Take care."

As I write these words almost a year later, tears roll down my face. The shock, disappointment, hurt and so much more remain, though my feet have been walking in his reality for the past ten months. The mourning for every dream and every expectation is not something that is done quickly.

Bald is a state of mind...

The day I got my hair, my head was covered.

At that moment in time, I would take my shirt off for anyone who asked me to, but my head would remain covered. On this day, I took a friend and we drove down Highway 4 to pick me out some hair. In the car, as the sun shone in on the passenger side, I explained that no one had seen me bald. I didn't even want to see it myself. The one piece of my body that was still private.

I had birthed three girls, so I knew the routine of taking off my pants for exams and deliveries. For the last two months, I had begun taking my shirt off for doctors and nurses and techs. One doctor would not even close the exam room before she had me strip down in front of her. No matter who was in the room: friend, family or acquaintance. Bare breasts were routine.

My head was my own. My final stand.

Yet on this trip, I knew I would have to release control. My hat must come off in order for a wig to be put on. My friend would know my secret. She would witness my last moment of privacy. I told her this, as I quietly cried.

We walked into a room of kind older women whose purpose for three hours a week was to outfit bald women, like me, with hair. I was by far the youngest woman in the room and my assistant had a hard time finding hair for my generation.

But we did it. It was not my natural color or length but it worked. I put it on and it worked. It felt right and I felt good.

We walked out of the room and I headed to the bathroom. Wearing my new hair for the first time. I checked myself out in the mirror, self-conscious, but smiling. It was a moment. I was empowered. The gift of normalcy, of fitting in.

A woman entered the bathroom. She probably caught me checking myself out. In my hand, I held a bag with a head for the wig to rest on. We were only five feet from the room that hands out such gifts to women.

She said, "Your hair looks very nice."

"Thanks," I said.

"What made you lose your hair?"

"Breast cancer," I replied.

"My hair won't grow very long either. This is as long as it will get. It has been this way for almost a year now."

I nodded and smiled. Being visibly sick is a blessing and a curse. People see you — see you differently. If they have a story that in any way aligns with yours, you will hear about it. Some stories are nice, comforting. You walk away feeling bonded. Many people have walked this road. Each has a story. Theirs can encourage you. Surely, I can be stronger than some of them! If they can get through it then I can too.

Some stories are terrible. Not at all what you want to hear. Those stories seem to gush from strangers. It is hard to hear the story from the other side. The stranger may be saying, "Someone I loved, who was very young is gone. I had planned to spend many beautiful vacations with and share many bottles of wine while watching the sunset with her. And as I stand here and see you, I am reminded of my love for her and I want to give you a bottle of wine in her honor." But what I hear is, "A young mom with kids like yours, didn't catch her cancer early either. She was your age and died leaving young children who may not even remember their mother at all. She never watched the sunset with them or me because we were too busy. You REALLY need to drink a lot of wine to get through this, but, oh yeah, you aren't allowed to."

This woman's story wasn't about a loved one or cancer. It was about a health problem that kept her hair from growing. That was our common point.

So, as I stood in the bathroom, still in front of the mirror, with a styrofoam head in my hand, she started talking to me about the empowerment of women.

"There is nothing for you to be embarrassed about. You are a strong woman with cancer. Your head is bald but you can be proud of who you are, and where you are at this moment. Life is about being honest with yourself and others. You can be boldly, baldly, beautiful. So, don't hide behind your wig."

"Thanks," I said, and I exited the bathroom, smiled at my friend and headed off to lunch.

At lunch, my hair felt strange brushing up against my face and neck. It had only been a couple weeks since I had hair but it already felt foreign. I felt confident at lunch in the nicest neighborhood and walking past all the high-end stores. We had such a good time we went out for dessert after lunch. The wig didn't itch or hurt. I never really thought about any discomfort. I would check myself out in every window reflection and think how nice it is to have permanent highlights and bangs that will never need to be trimmed.

That bathroom chat, though, stole some of my joy that day. There was no way I could have walked past shops and eaten lunch in the town, bald-headed. It wasn't going to happen. Men go bald gradually, and if you go bald, that is how it should be. Instant baldness is not acceptable to the psyche.

Months later, I do acknowledge there is some truth in the bathroom chat. Hair is a state of mind.

When I am happiest, I wear my hair. I put on my lipstick and my hair piece. I stand tall. I go out for coffee. I call my mom. The hair doesn't make me feel that way. I simply want to look in the mirror and see a reflection of my heart.

When I am frustrated, and tired of feeling tired, I have absolutely no desire for hair. Nothing will make me more infuriated than the suggestion of wearing hair. I don't feel normal. I don't feel healthy. I don't want to be associated with those who walk whole and well. My body is broken and weak. I wake up and it is a fight to walk downstairs and a workout to walk up the stairs. I feel bald. I have been stripped of all that was previously taken for granted. I look at the calendar and see an endless round of treatments. I cannot grocery shop or even be left alone with my own children. Bald resonates with my heart. I am no longer who I was. I am bald. I am doing this, but don't expect me to do life in the same way I did before right now. See my head, all of me has been stripped away, I don't want to cover it up. I want to be real, for you to look at me and know how I feel. I am stripped bare, inside and out. There is no frivolity of the body or soul that remains. Bald is who I am.

ERICIA LEONARD Walking through mud...

It's about facing one's mortality while trying to keep the courage to continue on for your family. It's like walking through mud with high heels on. You slip and fall and then you get up and try again, over, and over and over. Sometimes you stay down for a while, sometimes someone throws you a rope to help, but the mud is always there and the journey is never-ending.

How long can one go on knowing they will never make it out of the mud?

How many tears can one person cry from watching their family struggle from the other side?

You hear them cheering you on and that's what keeps you going, but no matter how hard you try to not think of it you know you will never make it

OUT OF THE MUD!

MELISSA ZIEMIAN I also feel very strongly about positive thinking...

My oncologist last November said I'd be lucky to make it to Christmas. I planned my funeral because of the power of this doctor's words. I started receiving Reiki weekly in my home and changed my mindset dramatically. This without a doubt strengthened me to start fighting again and resume treatment after two months of hospice.[12]

---

[12] Melissa died December 25, 2018

ERICIA LEONARD Good day today...

Great news from CTCA. All my tests came back negative for additional cancer!!

My oncologist actually talked to me and listened. Although I didn't exactly get every answer I was hoping for, I was able to get alternatives, different ideas, understanding, and most importantly a TEAM.

A few things we need to tweak and work on but all in all I received more Information in three days than I have yet through all of this.

I do have to see the neurosurgeon tomorrow for one more test, I'm scheduled to come back for follow up next month. I can finally say I'm starting to feel more excited if you can actually be excited to have cancer. I feel that I have hope and that maybe, just maybe, I can get my issues under control and get my life back.

DANIELLE WARREN The crushing words of terminal...

As Metastatic Breast Cancer patients, many of us aren't *sick*. We're among the healthiest terminally sick patients around. In fact, you might not be able to pick us out of a crowd. The scary part is that we might be stable and have no symptoms and suddenly, after major progression, we're moving into hospice. This can happen in DAYS, people!!!!!

I've seen it and it's a fear we all live with. The disease is so unpredictable. We're chronic until we're not.

Don't let anyone tell you you're a *forever fighter* or a *lifer*! Both imply the disease will be managed over our lifetime. They don't mention that our life is expected to last a scant eighteen to thirty-three months after an MBC diagnosis. Don't let anyone downplay the seriousness of the diagnosis, the finality, and the crushing effects of *Terminal*. THIS is MBC!!!

JEANETTE RHILE Stage 4 breast cancer is a terrifying roller coaster...

October 2017

Today was tough. Three months ago, the scans showed that the treatments were working. Now the latest scans show that the tumors in my liver are growing again. So next week I move on to a different treatment and wait for the next scan to see if it's working.

April 6, 2018

This week marks one year since I learned that the breast cancer has returned and spread to Stage 4. I haven't posted an update in three months because I haven't felt like there has been any new news, but in reflection, that is not entirely true. Every day that I wake up and get to go to work to help support my family is good news. Every day that I get to spend being a wife and mother is good news. Every day that I get to praise God and thank Him for His goodness and mercy is good news.

Physically, I must be exceeding expectations. When I told my oncologist last summer that my thirteen weeks of short-term disability would work out perfectly to get me through chemo and then I would return to work she quickly responded, "Oh, this is going to turn into long-term, you won't be going back."

What a kick in the gut! I chose to keep that to myself and not take her word for it. I have a different doctor now, thankfully. I'm choosing hope, not statistics! When I read about the *advances* in breast cancer treatments that are extending longevity by mere months, I know that my hope is not in what the oncologists have to offer. There's so much more to surviving this than just taking the prescribed treatments.

Here I am, a year later, working full time, getting a very tolerable treatment every three weeks, no further progression of the cancer, feeling grateful and full of Hope for a long and healthy life with my family. This cancer has been an odd gift, opening my eyes to the beauty in the little everyday things in life. Slow down, pause, savor it. Repeat.

I don't have this mindset nailed down yet, believe me, there are many times I have to yank my mind back from the hopelessness that lurks. It's a constant battle. But the more I pray for it and practice it the easier it gets. It's not that I fear death. I have a hope in Jesus that all the promised glories in heaven are waiting for us. It will be a wonderful place. I just don't want to not be here for my family. Even though we always talk about the kids growing up too fast, part of me is worried that it isn't fast enough. While it seems like my oldest is already on his way out of the nest, as he talks about college and career plans, and I'm thinking, "how can that be so soon, but yay, maybe I'll get to be here for him as he reaches that milestone." I want to see all my kids off to college or wherever they choose to go and be there for them as they find their paths.

Delaney is only eight, so I have a lot of years to keep hanging in there. The next scan is probably at the end of April. I'm expecting more good news then. Y'all keep praying because praise be to God, it's working. I thank God every day for all of you.

May 1, 2018

I just got the news that is trying so hard to steal my joy. The PET scan results I was given this morning are not good. The cancer is advancing again, no longer responding to the treatment. My oncologist has presented me with, now, the third line of defense that he has to offer, which is an oral chemo. Please pray that we will make the best decisions about the course of treatment and that regardless of the outcome, that I and my family can continue to find joy in every day and feel God's grace with us.

Without going through this, I don't think I would have ever had the courage to post a message like this... or had the mindset to truly, deeply, desire and seek a personal relationship with God. Perhaps that is the purpose in my trials, to lead me to this better place in my spiritual walk and encourage others to seek it as well. I want to give a special shout-out to Lynn Duy Moore for being that light for me in the workplace.

Thank you for your devotion to spiritually nurturing those around you. You have been a great encourager.

August 2018

Good news/bad news...good news is I was at my oncologist this afternoon and received the results of yesterday's PET scan, which shows all bone lesions have resolved and the liver lesions show mild improvement. Nothing looks like it has progressed, so the oral chemo that I've been on since May 1st appears to be working. Praise be to God!!

The bad news is, this oral chemo makes me feel like death and is the reason I was seeing my doctor today, to try to get some help with the severe dehydration. For a week now, I have been unable to eat much of anything at all and had vomiting and diarrhea beyond anything I've ever experienced. After coming in for fluids Monday and Wednesday, today the doc decided I should be admitted to the hospital for two days of some intensive re-hydration. So, once I'm mended, we will try to figure out some adjustments to dosing so I can stay on this medication and have some better quality of life.

My weekend at *'spa'* Novant Health will hopefully have me feeling well rested, nourished, hydrated and back to my old self so I can see the kids off to their first day of school Monday morning. Please keep me and my family in your prayers. I do feel them all and know that God is answering.

After Note: I was kept for three nights in the hospital and missed seeing my kids off on their first day of school. The life of a STAGE 4 MOM!

KEELI AYARS His only answer was, *Because I love you...*

Yesterday, after dropping his ten-year-old sister off at dance class, my five-year-old son and I headed off to Costco. We didn't have far to drive, but in that five minutes, Connor blurted, "I don't want my mom to die". It seems like that statement came from nowhere, but in our house, we live with a big, mean, elephant that is always in the room. Most moms can answer this statement with something like, "Oh, honey, I am not going anywhere", but I can't. I try to deflect. Unless I am hit by a bus, I know what I will die of, and I know it will be sooner than most thirty-six-year-old moms of kindergarteners.

I asked him why he would say that? His only answer was, "Because I love you." I had a hard time not walking into Costco with a face full of tears.

In the early spring of 2016, I went to my well-woman check. Everything looked good. I lied to her when she asked if I did self-breast exams. After all, I was thirty-three years old, not an age where breast cancer is a huge concern. A couple of months later, while watching TV, I absentmindedly rubbed a hand over my right breast. I felt a huge lump, the size of a ping-pong ball. However, even then, it didn't seem like a big deal. I had heard stories of grandmas and aunts getting lumps removed, I figured my family just had lumpy breasts. I would bring it up at my next well woman exam a year later.

When I finally did bring the lump up with my doctor, she was a little more concerned. Within a week, I found myself getting a breast ultrasound and a Mammogram. I was convinced that those results would be negative for cancer. I was thirty-four, a mom of two, doing well at my job and happily married. These things don't happen to people like me.

On Sunday, April 9th, 2017 my dad fell down our garage steps and broke his leg. I thought this would be the worst thing that happened to us this week. My dad is our *'manny'*, always helping around the house and with the kids. We depended on his mobility. However, this worry would be small compared to the phone call I received the next morning. It was Monday, April 10th, and I was sitting at my computer in my home office working away. When the phone rang, it was the doctor's number. I assumed the call was to tell me that my test results were in and there was nothing wrong with me. What the doctor did say changed my life.

"Hello Mrs. Ayars, we are sorry to tell you that the test results were carcinogenic."

There is a lot to unpack in that statement. First, Mrs. Ayars is my mother-in-law. In thirteen years of marriage, I do not believe I had even once been called Mrs. Ayars. Also, the word *'carcinogenic'*, I have heard that in anti-smoking commercials but never in reference to anything that could happen to me. But by the end of the day, I had an appointment to meet with a surgeon.

When we met with a surgeon, he urged us to do a genetic test. I thought that the results of this test would determine whether I would do a lumpectomy, a single mastectomy or double mastectomy. I still thought it was something I could cut out and be done with.

It was because of this hope, I still went on a business trip, I was not about to let this interrupt my life. During this trip, my back started hurting. I was sure that I had picked up my son wrong and the pain was compounded by sitting in an airplane and airport for hours at a time. By the weekend, I was back at home in Denver, my back hurt so bad I couldn't breathe. Since I was seeing an oncologist the next day, I would ask him for some painkillers. However, when I mentioned this to my new doctor, he was a little more concerned. He ordered an MRI. I was irritated. I was sure this was just a coincidence. He also ordered six rounds of strong chemotherapy and a years' worth of targeted therapy. This was a shock to me. I thought we were just going to cut this lump out. My diagnosis was starting to get more real. I was going to get sick. I was going to lose the long curly hair I had always been known for. I thought at very least my summer would be awful. I didn't know how much worse it was going to get.

A few days later I arrived for an MRI. I was annoyed when the hospital collected $700 from me. I was sure that this was a waste of time and money, after all, I was sure my back pain was unrelated. In my mind, it was just a pulled muscle, it would go away with rest.

On May 9th, 2017, I arrived at the Cancer Center for my first round of Chemo. I showed up ready to be a badass cancer fighter. I had my adult coloring books, laptop with movies, pillows, and blankets. I just had to get through the preliminary doctor's appointment. I should have known, when along with my husband and I, the doctor, physician's assistant and two nurses came into the small exam room. I don't remember the exact words that were used but I remember their impact. The MRI showed that there were *numerous* tumors on my spine. This result meant that my cancer had gone from a curable Stage 2 to a deadly Stage 4. The median prognosis for Stage 4 breast cancer is three to five years. It may be slightly better for me because I am young, and the metastasis was to bone and not to other organs. However, I was no longer eligible for surgery. Surgery is to stop cancer from spreading, once it has, there is no point to this effort.

I was given a private room to take my first round of chemo. There was a bed that I was able to lay in and cry. I cried for all of the things I am likely to miss. I have a daughter. Am I going to miss her trying on her first prom dress, her moving up to college and her wedding? Will I miss my son playing little league sports? Who will play Santa for him? What will he be like in middle school?

Now that the strong chemo is over, my life has changed. I tried to go back to work, but I will be leaving in a couple of weeks. Chemo Brain is real, I find that I do not have the same problem-solving skills I had before chemo. I get tired quickly, I get sore quickly, I get sick quickly. I am able to do small things with my kids, like go to Costco. However, I am dependent on my husband for any chores that require driving more than fifteen minutes. I am also not able to immediately comfort my children when they worry about losing me. Our priorities have changed. We take more vacations, worry about little things less. I am trying to make their childhood rich with memories and love. When they look back on me, I want them to remember the fun we had, not the illness.

KAREN BYRNE There's so much I didn't say...

From the diary of Karen Byrne:

In March 2016, I felt a lump in my right breast. I'm not a hypochondriac, but in my heart, I knew it was cancer. I had been having occasional pain in my armpit and in a few seconds, as my head was spinning, I knew it had spread. I saw my gynecologist first, and she recommended the Anne Arundel Breast Center to me. What a blessing...the place is great!

In April, I had mammograms, biopsies, ultrasounds, and an MRI. It was cancer and it had spread to my lymph nodes. I was scheduled to have a double mastectomy at the end of May then radiation and chemo. Doug and I sat down with our three kids, Jackie, then sixteen, Chloe twelve and Derrek six, to tell them about the cancer and what to expect from treatment. Derrek thought it was very cool that I would be bald. Someone asked him if he would shave his head, too. He responded, "No! I don't want to be bald like BOTH my parents!"

I began having major swelling in my right arm. Blood vessels were bursting everywhere and the pain brought me to tears. I was admitted to Anne Arundel Hospital where the main concern was a blood clot. It turned out there was no clot, but tumors in my lymph nodes were compressing nerves and blood flow.

While I was there, the results came in from my CT and bone scans. The cancer was in my bones, my hips, spine, legs, ribs and more. At my first clinic appointment with my oncologist, Dr. Garg, he explained that the plan was changing. No radiation or chemo and since the cancer had already spread, a mastectomy wouldn't benefit me and we had to *take the battle to the blood.*

I started Tamoxifen since my cancer is hormone positive. The goal was to starve the tumors and lesions on my bones. He prescribed therapy on my arm. I was wrapped up tight and had lymph node drainage massage three times a week for six weeks. My arm felt much better and I honestly felt pretty good physically. By summer, the shock of it all was taking its toll. I was just going through the motions of life and really wasn't enjoying it. Dr. Garg prescribed Effexor and it was a life-changer. I felt better almost immediately. Just in time to enjoy a dream vacation gifted to us by Leslie's Week, who gives vacations to Stage 4 breast cancer patients and their families. My family spent a week at The DreamMore Resort in Pigeon Forge, TN. They spoiled us. We all had an amazing time.

I returned to work in September and for a while, the scans always showed improvement and I felt pretty good. I don't know if bone lesions hurt worse when they die, but I know that my body hurts, especially my hips. I battle that daily. In November 2016 I had a hysterectomy and the doc put me on Letrozole and Ibrance, which costs over $13,000 for twenty-one pills. Thank God for insurance!

The hysterectomy threw me into full blown menopause and holy hot flashes! I have fans everywhere. It's getting better. Scans were steadily showing improvement until May 2017 when two tiny spots showed up in my liver. We are watching them. In July 2017, a huge *something* appeared in my lung. We thought it was an infection because it didn't appear on the scan to be cancerous and I had been sick and coughing up all sorts of loveliness. I took an antibiotic and soon felt great. At the beginning of September, I was getting winded easily and felt like crap. My oncologist was worried it was a blood clot and thankfully the CT scan revealed pneumonia.

For the last month, I've just been trying to catch my breath! It's now the beginning of October, breast cancer awareness month. I spent the day getting a CT scan and a bone scan. I will see Dr. Garg on Wednesday to go over the results. I'm curious if the huge *thing* is still in my lung, why I am still having trouble breathing? Have the two spots in my liver grown? Waiting for results is the worst.

I know this was long, but there's so much I didn't say. How this affects my family, job, future plans, etc. will have to go into another post. Stay tuned![13]

ERICIA LEONARD
Today was a hard day...

Today was a hard day. The day before this was worse. But as my crappy day continues, I see little things to make me smile like listening to *The Grateful Dead* and playing board games with the kiddos.

Depression is a horrible, horrible side effect. I ask myself, "Am I good enough? Do I do enough? How much can I cram into one day? Have I taught them enough?"

The pain makes it so hard to get through the day but without meds, I can't function.

I wish my anxiety would lessen just a little bit! But until then I'll take the little moments of happiness because that's all I have to hold on.

Feeling nervous...

I leave today to go back to Philadelphia, seems like I got home yesterday. I have back shots and pre-administration testing Wednesday. Easy rest Thursday and Gamma Knife on Friday at 5:00 AM.

One of the reasons this took so long to coordinate was because I need both the

---

[13] Karen died on May 10, 2018

Gamma Surgeon and the Neurosurgeon to work together on this because the new tumor is located behind and deeper than where they did brain surgery and there is still a fair amount of swelling. Gamma Dr. also said that because my cancer is so aggressive and I "seem like a no bullshit woman", that when he is there and if he sees anything more, even tiny, he's going to zap the crap outta them lol.

Because I fell three times in Philadelphia, I now have my grandma's old purple cane that I might bedazzle while I'm there cause, why not? After two weeks I will then start the million dollar meds that pass through the blood-brain barrier and will help seek and destroy all future (*if any*) brain tumors and any other cancer tumors too. This is a lifelong type of chemo treatment that may or may not have the same side effects as chemo — hair fatigue, etc. It is an immunization suppression drug which means Lysol, Purcell, and all that. I will ask that if you are sick to stay away. My mother will be with me for this trip and I have a feeling it's going to be hot chocolate and Christmas movies.

Another hard day...

Update the mummy wrap fell off during my whole three hours of crap sleep. Going to see if I can get it re-wrapped. Notice the almost black eye which is now swollen. BUT the process of Gamma was completely different this time. More invasive, more painful, more difficult... that being said with lots of tears and serious anxiety I made it. This is going to be it, I have some positive thoughts on this. I start my new meds in two weeks. The process will start all over but screw cancer...fight, repeat, fight, repeat!!

LISA COOPER QUINN I am tired of...

If you get tired of seeing my posts about Metastatic Breast Cancer, I'm sorry but I won't be apologizing for all of them. I'm tired, too.
I'm tired of seeing my friends die.
I'm tired of so little money going to fund true research.
I'm tired of all the pink ribbon propaganda.
I'm tired of companies making money off of my death and everyone else's.
I'm tired of looking at my children and wondering how much time I have left with them.
I'm tired of worrying about scans.

I'm tired of being worn out emotionally.

I'm tired of being worn out physically.

I'm tired of feeling like I can't make people care.

I'm tired of being afraid of dying.

SHELBY QUINLEY Another lump...?

I carried on during the fourteen years of being "cancer free" to have a wonderful husband and two of the most amazing kids ever!!! But in 2017, I noticed another lump in the same breast area.

I returned to my surgeon who performed the mastectomy. He scheduled an MRI, CT and PET scan. During the MRI I could see the scan and saw the highlighted spots and knew that I was in trouble. My concern was later verified when my surgeon called me while I was at my son's baseball game. He knew I was at his game and asked if he could give me some news. I had been waiting for this phone call for two days. He told me, "You have metastatic breast cancer." He told me *we* had some work to do.

My cancer had metastasized and returned in my lungs and bronchial area. I went to a breast cancer specialist at Sloan Kettering Memorial for a complete work-up. The doctor there contacted my oncologist in my hometown and they both worked out a regimen of treatment for me. I was so happy to hear that we were all working as a team — the two doctors, Dr. B and Dr. P, are two of the most amazing men and I consider them my family.

Following that diagnosis, I had six rounds of more chemotherapy followed by maintenance drugs on a continuing basis. My biggest reality hit me when I kept asking my oncologist probing questions about timing etc. He looked at me and said, "I am not a person who talks negatively but this will kill you". That's when it really hit home.

Damn, I have a husband and two kids. What in the hell!!! "Cancer, you don't know the bitch you are dealing with."

Anyway, life goes on.

WENDY MARIE

Pink isn't pretty, it's not a ribbon and it definitely doesn't help us...

While the majority of people believe that Breast Cancer is a pink ribbon, a pink pom-pom, a pen with a pink ribbon, a tote with a pink ribbon, an end-cap at your local Walmart engaging you to be a *part of the cure.*

First, a hard reality, you are not being part of the cure, you're just throwing your money away to propaganda, uniforms for NFL cheerleaders and kiosk after kiosk with items from handbags to Ziplock bags. It's all a hoax. They are not trying to fight the cure. Most of their funding goes to advertisement and six-figure CEO salaries. And when I asked for help, I wasn't given any, DENIED. Denied by the very people who claimed they would help me in their *advertising.*

A pink ribbon isn't the men and women fighting for their lives with Metastatic Breast Cancer. I cannot comprehend how people are unable to grasp the simple concept that if you CURE Stage 4 you cure them all. It's that simple. You will not have to worry about dying because there's a cure if you get to that point.

Breast Cancer is often very sexualized. Showing models with fake scars, beautiful bodies, and breasts with the strap so perfectly dangling from her shoulder. That's not what Breast Cancer is. It's CTs, surgeries, amputations, biopsies, MRIs, X-rays, radiation, chemo, IVs, blood tests, fear, worry, hate, anger, confusion, sadness, loneliness, medications, check-ups, anxiety, depression, insomnia and pain. It's so much more than a pink Snickers bar because it *supports us*!

We do not receive free boob jobs. We have reconstruction. Expanders placed to stretch your skin to fit the implants, complications and tram flap surgeries. Sometimes our bodies reject the implants, some choose to go flat, some reconstructions are amazing and look fabulous, some look completely deformed. However, in no way did any of us receive a free boob job. We amputated them and had foreign objects placed in our skin to resemble the breasts we once had. We tattoo our nipples on, we get prosthetic ones, or we go without. But none of it was free.

Save the Tatas, Save 2nd Base, No Bra Day with a bunch of nipples poking out — in no way supports those with breast cancer.

This is what a lot of cancer really looks like! Pink isn't pretty, it's not a ribbon, and it definitely doesn't help us.[14]

---

[14] Wendy Marie Nowicki died on April 23, 2019

LAUREN HUFFMASTER The end...

For nine months I showed up, twice a month, then every week and then every day. I showed up, every time, to willingly hand over a piece of my identity.

I could make a list of everything I consciously submitted to this process. So many tangible sacrifices. I gave up privileges. I gave up my ability to recognize myself in a mirror and gave up days at the park with my girls. Yet at the end of the process, these aren't the sacrifices that are leaving me raw.

On the last day of my cancer treatments, I was not jumping for joy as you might think. Instead, I sat, quietly, with tears rolling down my face. Raw is the best way I know to describe the feeling.

I expected, as my strength returned, I would find myself as I was last November. Instead, I find myself changed. The landscape of my heart has been altered more than that of my skin. I feel as if I have shed an old identity. One that served me well but was not to be carried into a new era.

Here at the end, I realize I spent nine months focusing on the external changes and haven't spent enough time acknowledging the internal.

Now that the season has passed, life looks different. I look different. I feel different. And I am not sure how to start again.

DEANNA CHASE RAYMOND Update...

November 3, 2018

For those of you who are wondering and don't know what's happening to me here is an update.

I woke up Thursday morning feeling like I was having a bad dream where I was half asleep and couldn't wake up so I hit Shawn a few times to get him to wake me up. This happens a lot. He woke up and realized something was not right!

I was having a seizure but didn't realize it!! Shawn immediately dialed 911 when it first happened and then called my parents right away. They actually got there before the paramedics! Long story short, I was taken to the hospital where they did an MRI on my brain and found four tumors. Three are very small, one is larger and swelling, and that's where the seizure took place. They sent me home with tons of steroids for the swelling and gave me seizure meds.

I saw my radiation oncologist yesterday morning where we discussed seeing a neurosurgeon on Tuesday plus brain radiation! After I see him on Tuesday, they will get me set up for the radiation on my brain. I was told five, maybe to ten, treatments! I had a PET done to see where else the cancer is. We know it is in my lungs, liver and now brain. But I need to see if it is anywhere else for determining treatment!

My oncologist called me and we discussed stopping my immunotherapy and starting chemotherapy after radiation! I will know more on Tuesday after I see all of my doctors and come up with a real plan! THANK YOU So Much, everyone, who has reached out to me and offered help. It is so much appreciated. For those of you wanting to help and not sure what to do please contact my mom Gigi Gerhardt.

Because of the seizure, I can't be alone so Shawn will be with me 24/7 and I can't drive! If you are wanting to help with anything, a meal or donation, get with my mom. She is coordinating them! Or if you have a gift card you would like to donate, or a card you want to send to me, you can bring it to the salon, or mail it.   Any help right now is so wonderful and I can't thank you enough for everyone who has helped or said a prayer for me. Thank you, Thank-you, Thank you!!! Just so you know I will not stop Fighting, Laughing, Loving, and Living my Life to the fullest! My family means the world to me and if not for myself I will do it for them!!

From: GiGi (DeAnna's Mom)
To: Jill Murray

Thank you so much, Jill. This is the hardest thing in my life. I keep it together in front of her cause she's my mini-me but inside I'm dying and watching my baby girl like this. I wish it was me with all my heart. You all at LESLIE'S WEEK were so good for her. She had an amazing time and met so many great friends. Y'all are truly amazing women. Thank you for your meal advice. I'll look into it right now, I'm just coordinating through my friends and family. This small town is an amazing place. Everyone is pulling together like one huge family. I'm not sure if DeAnna told you, I do hair so I know tons of people here and they're incredibly kind to us. Thank you again for reaching out to me and being so kind and sweet to my DeAnna. Love to you!

From: Jill
To: GiGi

I pray for DeAnna. But I also pray for YOU and the family. It is heartbreak, that cannot be explained, to witness the suffering of someone we love and the helplessness we feel because it is all beyond our control. I do not have to know you to know your heart. My deep love and continued prayers. I pray for DeAnna's miracle. I pray for peace for her and all of you as you journey together. And I pray that you all feel the love and light sent to you by those you know and those you do not (like me), that it surrounds you and sustains you. You are not alone.

From: GiGi
To: Jill

Thank you, Jill, those words mean a lot to me we will fight always and never give up hope!!

December 2, 2018

Sorry, it took so long, I've had a lot going on. I finally got released out of the hospital on Tuesday and we came back home Wednesday. Thursday, I saw my oncologist. Yesterday I had a full CT scan and had chemotherapy! The scan showed a significant increase in my disease everywhere since the last one on November 2nd so we are pretty sure this chemo is not working and we have to move onto a very strong chemo named Halavan! We are not sure what it's going to do but I am very hopeful that it's going to work. I need as many prayers as possible for this to work for me!

It has the potential to make me very sick but everyone reacts differently and I am feeling strong enough to take this on. Ain't nothing gonna hold me down!! My babies need me and I am a fighter! The biggest concern is I have a very large mass in my liver that literally grew four times the size since the last scan only four weeks ago! Still, I am very hopeful and positive that this chemo is going to work — IT HAS TOO!

Thank you, everyone, for all the love and support. We need a lot of prayer and positivity right now and I just want to make this Christmas the best one ever!! This Thursday I start Halavan and will keep you updated as

I go!! Again, all the positive comments, and prayers, and love really help me get through my day. Thank you!!

Let's do this...I'm ready to kick this cancer where it belongs. Who's with me??

NINA MUELLER

December 4, 2018

Turning out guys it's been a great ride. Please take care. I am dictating this so bear with me. I'm having my last evening with my family. Thank you for being part of my life.

Know that I am at peace now. Be the best you can be and don't regret your decisions. I love you all. No one will be replying to this Facebook post, so please don't bother. Good night, my friends and family.

God bless you.[15]

DEANNA CHASE RAYMOND Update..

December 31, 2018

I had my second round of radiation treatments today!! Seven in total! Thank you, mom, for taking me! They are very exhausting!! On Wednesday I start the eighth treatment on the large tumor on my liver so I will be getting eight treatments a day for ten days straight which is eighty treatments of radiation!! Wish me luck and lots of prayers for strength and free of pain!!!!!

From GiGi (DeAnna's Mom)
January 2, 2019

DeAnna's hemoglobin is still very low after infusion so they are keeping her in ER overnight. There are no beds, they are full, they are gonna give her another transfusion and scans of abdomen and chest to make

---

[15] Nina died December 18, 2018

sure no obstruction etc. They're covering all bases. Thank the lord, prayers for our sweet beautiful girl, for comfort, answers, and make her feel better.

From: GiGi
January 7, 2019

DeAnna has been in recovery since 10:30 by my side. She's sleeping and did very well today. She has to lay still for hours then off to the oncologist at 4:30 for results from scans. Pray for some good news and relief from all the pain she endures on a daily basis!!! I hate to see her suffer but so happy to see her sleeping so well. First time in months since she's been on the steroids. Love my sweet beautiful girl. Thank you all for prayers and texts, love to you all. Also, want to thank our wonderful nurse, Dana, you're the best!

From: DeAnna
January 7, 2019, 7:48 AM

Good Morning everyone sorry I haven't been on Facebook to update Y'all. I have been in and out of the hospital the last week! I had 2 blood transfusions several scans and now am headed to get a procedure done called Y90 mapping that is followed by another procedure on Friday where they will inject radiation directly into my liver tumors! This is a very promising treatment and they think it should shrink most of my liver tumors because they are too big to do regular radiation at this point!

The five new tumors on my brain have doubled in size so we are planning on doing more pinpoint radiation while we are doing the liver radiation! Today we will see my oncologist about which chemo we will be starting and hopefully everything will work out as planned. I know it will because all you prayer warriors and God are by my side!! Thank all of you for praying for me and stopping by and just showing so much love and support!!! This procedure is gonna be very painful. Please keep me in your prayers!![16]

---

[16] DeAnna Chase Raymond died on March 14, 2019

DANIELLE WARREN

Shared a Memory
January 7, 2019

Three years ago, since I started my first chemotherapy. And now I'm almost 50 (January 16.) A lot has happened in three years...

I've lost my hair, most of my eyebrows.

I have dealt with some nasty, nasty chemo (Taxotere) that made me almost want to stop and give up.

I've done ten consecutive rounds of radiation to my L3.

I started with one oncologist.

Got a second opinion and found out I was on the right plan of action but I was missing a key component that I needed - a bone strengthener.

I have gone from having a CT and Bone scan every three months to every six months.

I took my health in my hands and got a different oncologist, one that knows where my cancer is.

And we now added an Echo in there every three months.

My hair is growing back, but not like it used to be.

I have had two port placements.

My body was medically pushed into menopause.

I had a hysterectomy and now not medically pushed into menopause anymore — it's FULL on HOT FLASH central here!

I have learned to make memories with the ones I love.

I have started to make a Legacy.

I have learned who 'real' family and friends are.

I have learned that it is up to you to be your own advocate. It may be scary.

But if you want to be here for your family, friends, and kids, make sure you do what needs to be done. That is exactly what I am doing and will continue to do!

And through all of this, I have gained friends, Metasisters and Brothers, lost friends, and have been shown that I can Thrive with Metastatic Breast Cancer.

And most importantly, I've learned that it isn't a bad thing to be stubborn, have a backbone and tell it how it is. This is me. And that's not going to change.

Three years going and many more to come!

RHONDA HOWELL Bad news...

January 10, 2019

I have been trying to find the words to tell everyone the news from my Oncology appointment yesterday. There is no pretty way to say it. My cancer is growing and it is not stable. This means I am officially off the most recent oral treatment that we tried, as it, unfortunately, did not work for me.

The new palpable nodule on my neck is definitely a cancerous lymph node. My liver tumors have grown and there is a new tumor in my liver. The cancerous lymph nodes in my abdomen also grew. Although I suspected progression due to my high tumor markers, the new palpable nodule on my neck, and the fact that I have been sleeping ten to twelve hours per day, this was obviously not the news we were hoping for.

My oncologist presented us with a couple of options. All of the options involve immunotherapy. The two options that would allow me to stay local also include IV chemo. Which unfortunately means I will lose my hair. The third option involved traveling to Nashville, TN weekly for at least eight weeks for a Phase I trial. My oncologist and I agreed that this was not our first choice for my next treatment.

I will be having a liver biopsy within the next week. Then, I will start IV chemo within the next one to four weeks, depending on which treatment option we go with. Please pray for us as we process this news. Thankfully our precious son has taken the news well so far.

Stage IV breast cancer is ugly, at times extremely painful and overwhelming. I am leaning on God to carry me through this storm.

January 11, 2019

Kelly began her chemo in November 2018 and it will continue until March 2019. When I asked my daughter, Kelly Prescott, for an update about her experiences going through chemo this is what she wrote on Dec 31, 2018.

"Chemotherapy is a life-saving medicine, no doubt, but it can take a severe toll on your life in the meantime. The chemo is making me vomit non-stop. I have lost thirty pounds. I have been prescribed a steroid Dexamethasone that I can take at home, in addition, a Sancuco patch to wear for seven days and two more pills called Emend I take the day after and the third day. I also continue to take Zofran and Compazine. They put off my fourth chemo for one week because I can't get the vomiting under control. I also developed an infection in one of my incisions, and that means even more medicine. I spent $235 dollars at the pharmacy today. It is a crazy expensive nightmare that shows no signs of abating and seems to put you on a highway that never ends.

I am still trying to work, as I need my insurance, and my family needs my income. It is a nightmare driving to and from work because I'm worried I will vomit or pass out. I am also worried about that happening at work. I already fell on the way to my car.

The danger of severe dehydration and infection is a constant daily threat. Bedridden for days can send you on a downward spiral. A trip to the ER and one to a critical care facility following chemo sessions helped to revive me. Unfortunately, that is only a temporary respite as chemo brings me right back to the same condition again.

Cancer brings up many mixed emotions. My *altered normal* is a place I would never choose to visit much less live there. So this is chemo — hours-long infusions followed by *side effects*. At first, its mild nausea, vomiting and hair loss then the malaise begins. That feeling of discomfort, illness or uneasiness begins and will soon become a constant companion. One day I'll feel great and the next so exhausted I can't get up. Just when I start to have more energy, another treatment brings you down again and is usually worse. I feel physically and mentally exhausted the majority of the time. My emotions are all unpredictable and shadow my every waking moment. Fear is my constant companion as I journey through chemo. Yes, chemotherapy is a life-saving medicine, no doubt, but it can take a severe toll on your life and that of your family.

I am so grateful for the prayers, the emotional support and the monetary gifts I have received. Every single one helps me in so many ways. I thank you for your continued support. God Bless you all."

ERICIA LEONARD Different days ahead...

My first year anniversary approaches of being diagnosed with Metastatic Breast Cancer that has now spread to my brain. So has my anxiety and issues.

To date, I have had several seizures due to the tumors swelling. This has resulted in 3 Gamma Knife (*pinpointed specifically targeting the tumor*) procedures and emergency brain surgery to remove one tumor, only to find out another was hiding behind it. The doctors have put me on a new chemotherapy pill that is able to pass the blood/brain barrier. Traditional chemotherapy cannot do this.

I have lost my ability to work, drive and most recently I developed steroid myopathy, which is a condition that happens when you are on steroids too long. This has caused me to lose muscle strength to the point where I have to use a cane most days. I have very little strength in my arms and almost none in my legs and thighs. I have swelling like most people on steroids, but ten times worse. I don't just have a moon face. The swelling goes down my neck, which causes me to choke on food and have trouble breathing. My neck, shoulders and even my back and part of my head are all swollen. I don't want to sound vain but I hate going anywhere because people stare, not just a glance, but long-standing like *"whoa"*. The doctors have reduced my steroids. I have been ordered to start immediate physical, occupational and speech therapy along with a visiting nurse. The doctors are afraid of me having another seizure and don't want me to be alone for more than a few hours.

I have not worked since the last seizure, which was approximately Thanksgiving 2018. Getting used to that plus not being able to drive was and still is hard. Mostly not driving as we are a busy family.

I'm trying to stay positive, but most days I feel numb and I am in pain. Other days I sleep all day. Taking a shower is an hour event because of how slow I have to go. I do have good days and I'm trying to stay motivated to do therapy because I know that it will help. My goal is to get better so I can be there for my family. I miss seeing my kids games. I miss spending time with my husband. I miss seeing my family and friends.

Visiting nurses! I never envisioned having to have nurses and therapists come to my house. I never thought about grab bars, raised toilet seats, shower chairs, baskets full of medication. Hell, I just turned forty-one. But here I am.

So, as different days lie ahead, I sit and wonder how much time I have before I get *better* hoping it's soon. I also wonder how much more time I have before I need the medical beds and wheelchairs and the nurses on a constant basis.

March 13, 2019

I wish I could be that woman who takes the cancer journey and turns it into this positive experience. Don't get me wrong, I have my good days and my bad days, but my so-so, blah days take up most of my days. I really appreciate positive people and hope that before I die I can become one of those people instead of being in this constant roller coaster of emotions.

I'm finding that not being able to drive due to my latest seizures has really taken a toll on not just me but my husband as well. He's a rockstar but we all get exhausted. Thank goodness for other girls that help take my older children to practices as well as my in-laws. I can see how much I took this for granted and how it has affected my family.

It will be four years July 2019 since this started and one year since being diagnosed with Brain Metastasis. In one year, I have had emergency brain surgery and three, soon to be four, Gamma Knife Radiation surgeries and a new immune therapy cancer drug that passes the blood-brain barrier which is fantastic. However, the side effects mimic chemo and I am having issues with side effects, nothing too huge, just annoying. My bad days come from just when I feel better and feel like I can handle my *new normal*, I have to have yet another procedure. When does it end?

Due to the massive brain swelling with the tumors, I have been on steroids for a long time and I have developed something called Steroid Myopathy. This has robbed me of being able to walk without a cane. I can't lift anything; my hands are so weak that I drop everything. I have swollen so massively that even if I could go out people stare and I have lost what little self-esteem I had left. PT, OT, visiting nurse and speech therapy has been ordered, but I might never lose the swelling. I had no idea that something that has helped me not to have seizures could have such consequences. And to make matters worse my husband won an all-expense paid trip for two to a Cancun Mexico resort, but due to the gamma and the pain management of this steroid myopathy/ PT/OT, we just don't feel comfortable going. I personally think I could have rescheduled treatments but my wonderful husband is worried and wants me to be able to enjoy myself and not worry about gamma side effects or walking around with a cane.

I guess there is a possibility we could go in November. My first thought was what if I die before November? How morbid is that? But that is my world now. I find myself getting rid of things. Trying to clear out crap that I have accumulated over my forty-one years. All the while ignoring what is more important, like writing letters and things like that to my girls. I just can't bring myself to do it.

I have to find someone to take me to a funeral home so I can look into options. I don't know who to ask? I don't want to ask family but I don't want to hide anything either. I just watched something about how traumatic it is on your body to be resuscitated. I had no idea and now that I'm terminal do I really want that? Questions, questions, questions. My head is spinning.

I had high hopes of going back to LESLIE'S WEEK to give back, now I find myself wondering if I can make plans for a week at a time just because I have no idea how I'm going to feel. I feel like I'm letting my friends, family and my cancer family down. I dunno, maybe it's the dreary weather but something has to give. I'm not ready to give up but I totally can relate to people who just say *"enough"*. I will continue to fight for my children and my family.

SANDRA GUNN How do they do it?

These women, how do they do it? How do they endure the unbearable pain? How do they endure the uncertainty of the return of cancer day-after-day for years? How do they overcome the loss of self-image in their disfigurement and the reflection they see in their mirror? How do they continue to live with optimism and love for all who surround them? Their courage is unfathomable. They are not Ordinary. They are Extraordinary! There are no women like them. There are NO women like THEM!

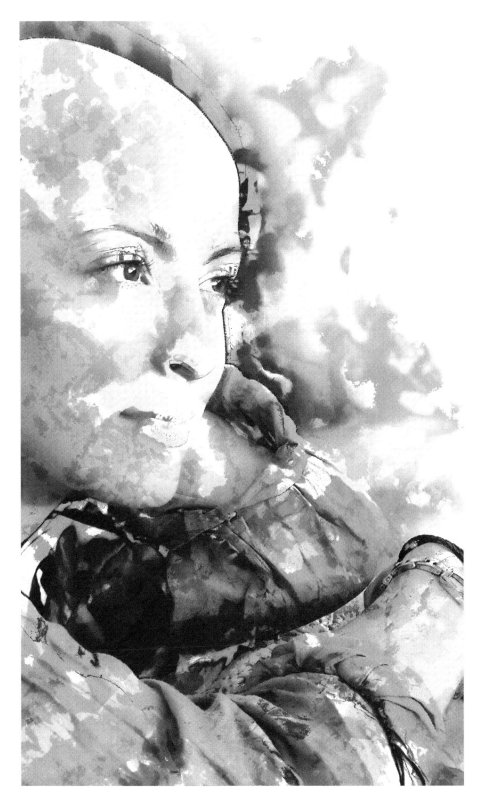

04. LAUREN HUFFMASTER
My Cancerversary

THIS IS THE ANNIVERSARY of my cancer diagnosis, my second cancerversary. In honor of this moment, I want to serve others by taking time to reflect on where I am emotionally and physically, and what I have learned this year. I hope my reflection is relevant to those who are learning to embrace survivorship and helps those newly diagnosed to not feel alone. I hope these thoughts will help us face what is ahead, with greater strength.

I spent this year learning to function within my new limitations. The things I have not done since Chemo — well, those pathways in my mind are gone, even if I did them 1000 times before cancer. So, whenever I meet someone new or try to solve a problem or remember a book I once read, I am stopped. Words evaporate and my brain is blank. The archives of my mind run like a slow computer.

I spent this year adjusting to scars. I am covered with scars. Scars that itch, and then bleed when I scratch. Scars that span from one side of me to the other. Scars that send shocks of pain, while retaining no other sensation.

I spent this year learning to limit the stress in my life.

I spent this year learning to manage my emotions. I cry under any pressure at all.

I spent this year learning how to empathize. I feel other's suffering, especially others with cancer. I hear of a mom with breast cancer and I am brought to tears, though I have never met her. I don't want anyone to walk this road.

I spent this year wondering who I should be. I, like most every survivor I have ever spoken to, struggle with the idea that now that there is hair on my head, I should feel normal. I don't. I have only begun to heal. My life is raw. Like the skin on my body, I seem to be paper thin. Too thin to withstand the abrasions life brings my way.

I spent this year with a cancer filter. Every new pain in my body creates a flashing alarm in my mind, alerting me to the fact that perhaps there is new cancer growing. Every mistake I make sets off a chain reaction of fear that the chemo damage will never heal, I will never recover. Walking into a doctor's office is an ominous experience. The smell of the building, the view of the magazines on the table, or the taste of the water fountain creates a blaring warning that something bad is coming or may be already present. These alarms do not resonate like polite cricket-like clocks but rather blare deafening alerts that I must manually reset within me before I am able to respond to the receptionist or answer a doctor's question.

I spent the year training my body and mind to not sink into that type of fear.

This is where I am, an honest look at me and my struggles. Though I cannot escape these experiences, I have set my heart on something different. Walking in this season has created a heightened sense of life and many transcendent moments, because of the presence of fear. I would argue that there are two types of fear, good fear and bad. Secondly, the best way to fight bad fear is to replace it with the good. As I minimize my natural fear, the kind that sets off alarms in my mind and stops me from moving forward in life, I am able to make space for good fears which come from taking risks, walking in hope, and stepping out in faith.

Let's take a look at good fear. We remember with great detail, a first date. Why do we remember it so well? Fear. We are scared of rejection, scared of making mistakes, scared our breath smells bad, just plain scared. Yet when all is said and done, fear makes the moment better. It gives us awareness of every detail. It locks moments into our memories with accuracy. It heightens our emotions. In essence, fear provides the capacity for us to feel emotion in a big way. In the right time, fear is a gift.

This same kind of good fear exists in sports, roller coasters, and adventures of every kind. We pay a lot of money to experience fear. We go to a scary movie, ride a roller coaster, climb up the side of a mountain, and paddle down a river because fear for a moment is exhilarating. Fear makes us feel alive. It drives out every other thought, focusing the mind, bringing joy and a sense of accomplishment. We love this type of fear and so we go in search of another ride, another river, another moment to hold onto. Unfortunately, these experiences are fleeting. We cannot truly achieve lasting peace or joy through back-to-back moments that expose us to good fear. Eventually, the ride won't feel scary and the river will be tame.

In our day-to-day life, we can experience fear by embracing risk. Risk means embracing something that has no guarantees and looking at the situation through a filter of hope. When we head out on the adventure, with no guarantees of what we will find, risk is there. Therefore, on our adventure, every experience is heightened.

Every memory locked in for a lifetime.

Why do we leave our house if there is risk? Because of hope. Hope is needed when taking risks. We set our minds above the problems that could arise. We hope for a beautiful day, despite the forecast, as we set out on a hike into the wilderness. We put our mind, our thoughts, and our faith in what is not readily evident. We embrace hope and put that hope into action through faith.

Unlike fear, these emotions are a choice. Unlike fear, the heightened sense of life that comes from hope and faith lasts for more than a fleeting instant. As long as we can hold onto our hope, clarity and peace remain.

Life with cancer does not on its own provide a fear that is good but it does create ample opportunity for hope and faith to thrive. In fact, in many ways, a diagnosis of cancer leaves a person with two choices. To live in involuntary fear, or to choose hope and the act of walking out that hope through faith.

This year I learned to hope in the strength of my body, in cures, in the kindness of people. I placed hope in love's ability to rise above. I placed hope in my ability to release all that I was and find something new, perhaps something better. I hope for these things. I have not found them and so I choose to walk toward them every day in faith. This risk, this faith, has raised my eyes above all that I currently am. It has given me a sense of calm in the storm. This hope has heightened my awareness of life. Like the experience of fear, living in a state of hopefulness and faith creates abundance in the mundane.

My year of hope has also gifted me an opportunity for clarity. Clarity is a common experience among cancer survivors, though we may not readily call it "clarity". Many of us have a sudden awareness of priorities, and how our lives align or don't align with those priorities. We actually experience joy when partnering with what we find valuable. Conversely, we carry an increased burden in the tasks that pull us from those things. We live with a sense of urgency. Do not waste the moment.

I would argue, this common experience is the result of hope in our lives. We are walking riskily. We are investing our hopes in things that we find valuable but cannot guarantee. We are experiencing faith, by choosing to adjust our lives to our hopes; by moving closer to our ideals every day.

Cancer gives us the ability to experience life like never before. Though it may not be the roller coaster ride we would have chosen, we are in fact on the ride of our lives. Though I see myself growing tired and emotionally weak, it is what I cannot see that keeps me strong. My eyes are set on all that I can imagine and hope for and I intend to keep walking in faith until these too are seen.

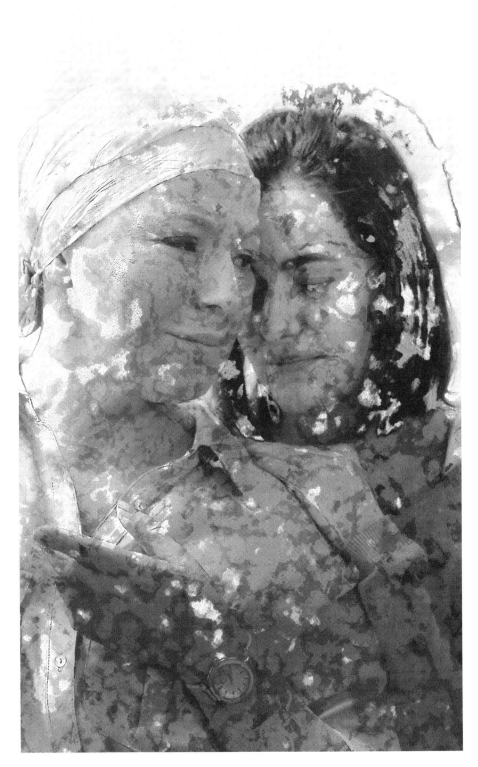

05. THE FAMILY
"She Has What?"

CHILDREN ARE BORN innocent. They have a creative spirit and yearn to exhibit their intensity and wonder for life. They are brought into their world by a woman. They are completely dependent upon her for their survival and nurturing. They cannot speak to her in a language. They can only communicate with her by sounds, gestures and reaching out with their small arms and eyes. They recognize her voice, her movements, and sense her faint aroma. She is the most important woman in their life and the most important woman they will ever meet.

The first woman children fall in love with is their mother. She is their treasure and they are hers.

It never occurs to children that she will leave. They think she is an invincible force and will live forever, or as long as they define forever in their childlike minds. When they are told, *"I have breast cancer"*, they have no frame of reference, no way to define the sadness and turmoil that will penetrate their lives. They are only accustomed to love, hugs, cuddling, games and family life, which does not include *cancer*.

Stage 4 Breast Cancer is a family disease. It impacts every member in astonishing ways. Many never understand its full impact until after it is over. Sisters, mothers, brothers, fathers, children, husbands, cousins, aunts and uncles are all changed. Their lives are never the same as before cancer. They carry a sorrow with them, a hole that is never filled again in the same way as before cancer.

These are The Families. These are their words of enduring the pain, the loss, and the sorrow.

CASON JONES Son (15 Years Old)
Hearing the cancer word...

I don't like to talk about this time, for all of us it is sad.

I am not good at expressing my feelings so this will be short. I had faith in my mom when she found out she had this cancer, she would OVERCOME IT!!!!!!! My mom is a warrior, she beat two other ones and I know she will beat this one too.

I guess you could say I lost my Pop, which was my mom's dad. He died from colon cancer about the time my mom was going through hers. Her dad was there doing the same thing, she really melted when she lost him cause she thought they would fight it together, but his body couldn't take the chemo. But as we all did we had to carry on and that is what she did.

I say, "God has my mom's soul but the devil will never have her spirit".

She is fighting the good fight and I know in my heart she is doing it with a vengeance!!!!!!!!!

JILL MURRAY Sister of Karen Byrne

Posted on Facebook
October 13, 2017

I usually think three times and type twice before I post. And this time it's been more thought and hesitation than that. But, I want to share a little about my sister Karen, my very best friend.

Karen decided to bravely share her personal MBC4 story a couple of weeks ago. I was so proud of her. Inspired by her vulnerability. In awe once again of her strength. There have been many times I wanted to post something and couldn't, it wasn't my story to tell. Her story is different from mine. She has Stage 4 Metastatic Breast Cancer and that's the lens thru which she now views everything in her life.

My story is that I witness and walk beside her on this journey and ride my own rollercoaster of emotions.

Karen is a better human than me. She is kinder, braver, funnier and closer to God. She has maintained an unwavering faith in His plan and I have many times loudly questioned Him, "Why?!"

Over the past 18 months many kind-hearted people have asked about her and in what I assume is an effort to be encouraging. They would mention things like, "She looks great! She's gonna beat this." But the truth, a truth I denied many times because it was too painful to speak, is: what it will take to beat 'this' is a

miracle! There is no cure. A Stage 4 Metastatic diagnosis is a terminal diagnosis. There are treatments to help keep cancer at bay but the average life expectancy after diagnosis is 33 months. Stage 4 usually 'looks good' because patients have passed the point of eligibility for all the poisonous lifesaving treatments.

When Karen sees her oncologist, the conversation is always versed around 'quality' of life. She may not look like she has cancer. But she certainly feels its effects. And when you love someone as much as I/we love her...my heart is broken. Broken! And it breaks a little more every time I allow my mind to view what is happening as reality.

People don't know what they don't know. And that's okay. But, what I want you all to know is that Karen is an amazing soul. Truly one of the best. I want you to know that she has faced many hardships in the wake of this diagnosis, physical, emotional, and financial. Yet she continues to smile and laugh and ask about someone else's day.

She reminds me of how blessed we are. We have such strong family bonds and with them, we remain encouraged and secure in the knowledge that we are loved. We know we never have to journey any path alone no matter how difficult it may be.

What I finally realized the other night while speaking to Mom and Pop was that some things are bigger than 'us' and that help needs to be outsourced. That although our love is strong, 'love' can't pay a bill. We are actively working on fundraisers to help alleviate the weight that Karen and her family are carrying. As soon as I have details, I will be sharing and I hope that anyone reading this will share also. Until then and always, all prayers and positive thoughts are welcome and appreciated.

Posted on Facebook
October 23, 2018

I haven't posted much in a long while. Most of my thoughts I feel are too personal to share. My head has been spinning for over a year. Facebook has never been my 'go to' when I have something to say.

Sharing for someone else in an effort to inform, to encourage, or to honor is easier than sharing for myself. But, I am reminded that there have been times I have shared for myself and the unexpected outcomes were encouragement for others.

After Karen passed away and her memorial services commenced, I felt paralyzed by grief. Silence has been safety, a place to try to hide from heartbreak. As if not speaking about it would somehow make the hurt pass over me. But what I am learning…denial only lasts so long and this pain will not suddenly disappear at some magical point in time. I must allow myself to trudge through it, to cry, to remember, to forgive, to feel, to share.

I will never miss her less. This will never hurt less. Because I will never love her less. The world is different in her absence. I am forever changed by this loss. There is no going back. Life doesn't work that way. I must learn to navigate forward movement with whom I have become.

I know I am not alone in these truths.

Thank you to friends that check-in. Thank you to the people that remain present months later because they know that the sadness we feel hasn't diminished and that many days it takes all of our energy to stand up and put our feet on the ground. You know who you are and your love and continued support have been oxygen on days that we feel we are losing our breath.

MICHELE THOMPSON Mother of Lauren Huffmaster
A Mothers Response to "A Sweet Fragrance"…

Glancing down at the ringing phone a smile spreads across my face as I look forward to the call from my oldest daughter, my friend, filled with discussion about my grand girls and California adventures. Instead, I answer the call that changes all our lives forever.

"Mom, I have cancer….yes, I am certain…l will be starting chemo and radiation and then a double mastectomy….it's a fast-growing aggressive type". The uncontrollable tears began to flow along with a heaving pain in my chest and disbelief. NO! NO! NO! Not my precious girl. She's healthy, eats well, exercises, never smoked, or took drugs or drank too much. She's lived her life so well! As days went by the disbelief faded into reality and that heaving pain remains ever-present. SORROW began its journey in my heart. Life will never be the same.

Cancer respects no person. Doesn't care what scars it creates, or the pain it inflicts, not to mention the fear. It affects every person who touches the lives of its victims. All victims of the disease suffer, family and friends. No one will suffer as much as cancer's physical host but all lives suffer.

As a mother, I want to fix it. Make it all better. Tell my daughter it will be alright. I FEEL HELPLESS. It hurts 24/7. I live and work in Tennessee. She and her wonderful family live in California. This distance is heartbreaking and difficult. Even when I get to visit, I have to leave her all too soon. It is never enough.

Cancer steals away so much. I feel like it builds a wall between us. In trying to make conversation, it's hard to not talk about it. So you endure small talk, avoiding the *issue.* You once had plenty to talk about without discussing cancer, but now it dominates your thoughts. The cancer patient is tired of talking about it or there's more bad news no one wants to tell. Family and friends want to know what's going on but are afraid to keep asking. I have struggled with this even with all the love in my heart. It is difficult to have free conversations and I feel like a failure. I want to know what to say to cheer or strengthen her.

Prayer! Prayer is the only real help I can give. I pray day and night for healing, new medicines, and a cure. I ask for relief from the pain and fear my daughter lives with every moment, both emotionally and physically. I wake from a deep sleep and before I am even aware, I am pleading with God to help us. Prayer is our only true weapon against cancer. I constantly choose to trust in our great God who holds this in His loving hands. Nothing can waiver my faith in Him. Not cancer, not death, not the possible loss of my child and all that lies in between. It is the only peace I can find.

Lauren, my daughter's name, by definition means "A Sweet Fragrance". She is just that, to those who know her. She and her husband have a beautiful bond, they are ONE. Her children adore her, and she is an awesome mother. I could never have dreamed of a stronger, wiser, more beautiful child. She is the sweet fragrance of her name. She has used cancer to reach others, to make unexpected friends, to grow in this deadly environment. She has joined support groups and even started a non-profit to ensure cancer patients have life-altering adventures that will inspire them to fight on. Using the time she has here on this earth, she isn't giving up, but rather making such a difference. The fact that she finds the strength to go on so boldly and productively has to be a gift from God. Thus, the prayers we offer up are being heard!

I'm not entirely certain what to write about. I know that the years we have battled cancer in this family have been fearful, destructive, painful and way beyond sad. Cancer is a thief that steals your life away even while you are living. Death is not the enemy when you have faith in The Savior. We are all on the path to Eternity. It is this journey towards death that must be endured, no matter the sorrow and fear. Cancer is a constant reminder that we are on that journey.

I am amazed and blessed to see a young woman like my daughter prepare so well for that possibility. She makes eternal memories, preparing her soul in case there is no cure for her.

I came into her kitchen during a visit last spring. I was only dreaming of coffee. The lights were off. I heard her voice weeping, softly singing out the song *"it is well with my soul."* It broke me as I returned to my room and wept. She is brave. She is strong. She is HIS. And she will always be my girl, my first born, my sweet fragrance.

PATRICIA JOAN MORGAN Mother of Kellie Prescott
A Mothers Response to Her Daughter's GoFundMe

My youngest daughter, Kelly, was recently diagnosed with cancer. She is a mother with children and grandchildren. Her husband is disabled and requires a full-time caregiver. Her seventy-one-year-old father came to live with her to help during the day. Kelly is the sole breadwinner of her household. Her health concerns began in 2015 with tests, biopsies, lumpectomies and lymph node removals. From 2015 through 2017 she was monitored closely and was still cancer free. Until...she wasn't.

Along with its hot, humid days, July 2018 arrived with a cancer diagnosis, and the beginning of a *new normal.* A biopsy and lumpectomy provided evidence of Invasive Mucinous Carcinoma in Kelly's left breast. Mucinous Carcinoma is an invasive type of cancer that begins in an internal organ that produces mucin, the primary ingredient of mucus. The abnormal cells inside this type of tumor are floating in the mucin and the mucin becomes a part of the tumor. This rare type of cancer can occur in any part of the body that produces mucin. It's more commonly found in the breast. Approximately five percent of all invasive forms of breast cancer have mucinous carcinoma present. Her first surgeon recommended surgery to remove the cancer and sentinel lymph nodes and this was performed as soon as it could be scheduled. The following month tests showed another surgery was indicated to get clear margins. That was unsuccessful.

In August 2018, Kelly decided to go to Cancer Treatment Centers of America in Atlanta, GA and began treatment there. A team was assembled on her behalf and surgery was scheduled for September 2018. A double mastectomy was performed and reconstructive surgery took place at that time. She was unable to work and was informed that she could place her name on a donated leave site at her office.

Following her double mastectomy, Kelly developed MRSA in her right breast and another surgery was performed the first of October 2018 to remove the expanders thus she could not proceed with the reconstruction. Once the type of MRSA was indicated she received antibiotics in preparation for her upcoming chemotherapy.

Even though she had a double mastectomy and began chemo on 11/19/18, she continues to work as she needs her medical insurance and a full paycheck. She travels about an hour to work each day and back home again. As the chemo progresses she may not be able to continue.

Cancer strikes and cares not if you have money for food, gas and lodging when your hospital is an hour away. It does not care about how much you may need to pay for the much-needed drugs. Prior to her cancer diagnosis, Kelly had endured lumpectomies, lymph node removals, and several operations to remove diseased tissue. Her doctor advises that the first half of the chemo should be tolerated well but the last half will cause mouth sores, hair loss, and lots of sickness and malaise. However, after her first chemo session, she was informed that she may lose her hair after two or three days as her immune system was severely compromised by the MRSA infection.

It is critical that I find help for my daughter, as she is the sole breadwinner in her home. And if the disease of cancer does not fully take you down, the medical expenses surely will.

JAYME FERRIS Sister of Danielle Warren
A Sister's Response to Stage 4 Breast Cancer

The day my sister sat us all down as a family is the day we received the heartbreaking news that my sister has breast cancer. It was one of the hardest things that I had to take in. I've never been so scared in my life when she told me. I tried to hold back the tears and stay strong but I couldn't. I had a million thoughts running through my head. Like, is she going to go into remission? Does she have a time frame? How are the kids going to be? Overall, I just didn't know what to think.

The day I went with her to her doctor appointment about the discussion of her double mastectomy and the implants was interesting about what was done, like how the silicone implants felt and, knowing you can get tattoo nipples. Everything started to become so real. I always thought, 'why does my sister have to go through this?' She's been through so much. She just lost her husband fifteen months before the indents appeared on her breast.

The day we all sat in the hospital getting ready for her to have her double mastectomy done was like, damn this is really happening. I had a million things running through my head. Will it be painful for her afterward? Can anything bad happen while she's in surgery? Is she overall going to be okay with how she looks? While we were waiting, the doctors came to her and made a change of plans. She was only getting her port to start chemotherapy and radiation because they found a spot in her L3. So it was a better option for her.

I definitely learned a lot throughout this whole thing. I'm so happy that she is maintaining the breast cancer and it hasn't spread anywhere else in her body! She is a tough woman and she will have a long life to live and will watch her two amazing children grow! Danielle, I am your little sister and will be by your side throughout everything and anything. I love you!

LINDA BREND Mother-in-Law of Danielle Warren
Three Years Have Passed

It is hard to believe that three years have passed since that frightful day that my daughter-in-law Danielle received her cancer diagnosis. We sat through one appointment where we prayed the lump would be just a harmless one. After all, she was only thirty something and had just lost her husband the year before. This could not be happening. She and the twins have been through enough, now this???

As we drove to the next appointment for a mammogram, we were still in denial that this would turn out to be the *C word*. We could not even say the word at that time. We sat through first the mammogram, then the biopsy, all within a couple of hours. We began to truly understand that this was not going to have the outcome we had been praying for.

We were so thankful we chose to go with Danielle for these appointments, we would never have let her go through all this by herself, even though she kept insisting that we go home, that she was alright. She is so strong as she has embarked on this unfair journey that was thrust upon her. She never complains about feeling crappy even though one has to assume she feels tired and filled with pain and all the other stuff that comes with receiving cancer treatments. She is always there for the many activities the twins are involved in, never giving in to the cancer.

We place her name weekly on our church prayer list and have many friends that continue to pray for a cure for this horrific disease. She continues to look at the bright side of things and this continues to be an inspiration to us and her twins. This diagnosis has changed us in many ways, but mainly we do not take anything for granted. We continue to be active in their lives and will always be there for whatever the future brings their way. We continue to pray for a cure for MBC for her and all those that deal with this disease.

Her husband is looking down from heaven and is proud of what she had done on her own.

KELLY SNETHEN Mother of Danielle Warren
A Mothers Total Disbelief

I have been pondering this for a few days. I was asked to write about my feelings when I found out that my daughter, Danielle, was diagnosed with breast cancer. The day I found out I was in total disbelief. I broke down and cried. I was really upset, this could not be happening, it wasn't fair. I was mad at God, Danielle has been through so much in her young life. How could God put more on her plate? She lost her father at the age of thirteen, lost her grandmother to breast cancer when she was four, both of her grandfathers to cancer, and she just buried her husband. All I could think of was how and why in the world did God think she could handle anything else? I wanted to know why her and why not me? Danielle is way too young to have to deal with this. I am older, I have lived my life. Danielle was just beginning to pick up the pieces of her life after her husband's passing and trying to get back to a normal life with her beautiful twins.

After her initial diagnoses in mid-November 2015, Danielle and I spoke several times about what she wanted to do and how she wanted to go forward. As a family, are we going to hit this head-on? It is Stage II breast cancer, okay what does that mean, a mastectomy? Has it gone anyplace else, cut them off and we will be done and everything will be okay?

Danielle and I sat in pre-op awaiting her seven to nine hour surgery. She was doing amazing and attitude was okay, I think the happy drug was taking effect. She was fine about losing her breasts just so the cancer was out of her. She felt they don't define who she is as a person. Just as long as she was going to be okay. Suddenly, the world stopped for us. Everything changed forever. Her oncologist and her surgeon walk in together and by the look on their faces, it wasn't good. The doctors said no surgery, it was canceled!

Danielle just had a biopsy of her L3, on December 31, 2015. She had a spot in her back that was giving her unexplained pain while she was at work. Danielle stared at the doctors as they were explaining, but I could tell she was in disbelief. She was lost. She wasn't sure where to go next. They explained that they wanted to start chemo immediately, the next day. Instead of the long surgery, they will be placing the port in for chemotherapy to start immediately. Her cancer jumped to her spine. Just the L3, the spot that was giving Danielle pain for months at work.

Thankfully she was already on her happy medicine because I am not sure on how she would have had reacted without it. Within weeks, she went from Stage 2 to Stage 4. It was Metastatic Breast Cancer. From that moment, Danielle and I were unsure what Stage 4 meant or what would happen going forward. We were both scared. I could see the fear in my daughter's eyes when she was in recovery. She wanted answers. I wanted answers.

Through this battle there have been a lot of ups and downs, her beautiful hair falling out, side effects and being sick from the chemo. There were moments she wanted to give up, wanted to stop chemotherapy! She was done having her kids seeing her sick, in bed, not being able to do everything that she could before Stage 4 breast cancer. She didn't give up. She knew what she was fighting for. She knew that her dad, grandma(s), grandpa(s) and husband were there through this and were giving her strength when she didn't think that she had it. She went through several rounds of radiation on her L3. There were mood swings, me not knowing what to do or say, me not knowing how I could help, and being upset that it wasn't me instead of her. I did not understand until recently that if anyone was sick they shouldn't be around Danielle.

Before her scans, Danielle freaks out. It is so hard to help her because I just do not understand what she is going through. I am scared to death! Danielle gets a little nasty at times but hell I don't blame her. She is scared. She is doing great with her maintenance chemotherapy and everything remains stable. I know this is not a guarantee but her being stable is all I care about.

I can't be prouder of her. She is a fighter for herself and also for others. She is a THRIVER! She goes to retreats and meets with others who are fighting this battle. Lately, she lost really good friends to Stage 4 breast cancer and that is very hard for Danielle. She not only fights for herself, or her boyfriend, she is fighting for her twins and she will not give up. She is trying to educate everyone about Metastatic Breast Cancer and I am so proud of her for doing this. She has given me so much information that I didn't know. She has shown me the strength that I wish I would have.

Danielle does not sit around but is doing everything she can with her children, making memories, and having fun with them. Make a LEGACY! They are 8 years old now and they know mom has cancer. They talk about it and her twins know cancer is not good and they understand when mom doesn't feel well. Danielle keeps that line of communication open with her kids. She wants them to know where she is going and why. She doesn't want them to wonder or worry more than they do. They are kids, so they need to enjoy life. That's what she does with them. Enjoy life to the fullest!

I hope this explains a little of what as her mother I am going through and trying to process with Danielle's diagnoses and her treatment for Metastatic Breast Cancer. It is so hard to put all of my feelings into words. I know that I am proud of Danielle and believe me I don't want to lose my baby girl to this horrible disease.

VICTORIA LEONARD (16 Years Old)
A Daughter's Response to Hearing Her Mother Has Stage 4 Breast Cancer

When I found out that my mom had Stage 4 cancer my first reaction was a pure shock, then hatred and fear. I had never thought that my family would be directly affected by cancer. I hated watching my mom go through everything that came with cancer. I hated feeling hopeless. I hated how this could happen to her and our family. I was angry — with life, cancer, the doctors that weren't fixing it fast enough, myself for being unable to help and I was angry at God!

Over the years I have learned to deal with the fear and my anger. I try to find the light in everything. I am now hyper-aware of the things I say to and about my family, how I interact with them and others. I enjoy spending time with my mom and try to help my parents out as much as possible. I also have a greater appreciation of the people who have helped us. It makes me happy to know that there are so many kind and caring people out there. I also see my mom in a new light. She is so strong and hopeful. She is amazing and I really can't imagine her not in my life. I know that she will beat cancer, she is a fighter. Cancer picked the wrong people to mess with.

TAYLOR LEONARD (15 Years Old)
The Hero Within Revealed
A Daughter's Response to her Mother's Stage 4 Breast Cancer

When I found out that my mother had stage 4 breast cancer and also metastatic cancer, it was a shock to me. I didn't know what to feel at that moment but all I could tell you is that I cried and cried and said to myself "why me" and "why my family" and hoping it was all a dream. Having my mom have cancer has been a challenge for me and my family. We had to face the fact that my mom couldn't do all the activities she used to do. The hardest part for me was seeing her in pain and not being able to do anything about it. But in every story, there is a happy ending, and mine was seeing her smile, and laughing through the hard times. Or all of us watching a show/movie together as a family.

My family and I have been through some dark times, and we're still not out of the woods yet, but I'm certain that if we made it then we can make it now!! Bob Riley said, "Hard times don't create heroes. It is during the hard times when the 'hero' within us is revealed."

Even though the past couple of years have been extremely hard for me and my family we had some amazing times together and this experience had made us even closer to one another. My mom is the strongest, bravest, most fearless women I know! And I'm not just saying that because she is my mom. It's the truth. This disease hasn't made her weak or made her feel like giving up. It made her stronger as a person.

DELANEY RHILE (9 Years Old)
A Daughter's Poem to her Mother's Stage 4 Breast Cancer

Try to read this without shedding a tear or two. Unbeknownst to me, Delaney wrote this and shared it at school today for cancer awareness day. Her PE teacher created a collage from my Facebook photos with the poem in the middle, laminated it, and sent it home as a gift. — Jeanette Rhile

My Mommy is a warrior, yes indeed it's true.

Most people had cancer once, but, my Mom's had it times two!

She has made it through the tough times, hair loss and regrowth.

But she has managed to keep a smile on during holidays and vacations both.

My Mommy is a warrior. She has her ups and downs.

And whenever I see her down I automatically frown.

She's sweeter than a gummy bear.

She's beautiful as the sun.

Don't think this poem's over yet, it only has just begun.

It all started when I was small, before our trip to Topsail Island where the air is fresh
and palm trees tall.

Turns out she had cancer, it was quite the bummer. Then she fights it off until last summer.

She got diagnosed with stage four, I had never felt so much sadness before.

My Mommy is a warrior. She is my inspiration, the sunshine of my rainy day.

She is the kind of Super Mom that always saves the day.

Despite all the bad times we still need to smile.

My Mom is strong and brave and for her, I'd walk a mile.

I love Mom.

LYNNE HENDRIX

A Poem from The Mother of Avery Harrison

A little background:

The Lord gave me this poem shortly after having my fourth miscarriage. I had started collecting angels, and one day I was out and about and came across a seraphim angel in a store on a clearance rack (these angels are generally quite costly). However, this one had a broken wing. As I looked at this gorgeous figurine the Lord spoke loudly to my heart, "a broken-winged angel still can sing!!!! I asked how much for her, the cashier told me that they could not sell it because of the damage. I asked what were they going to do with it and she said it would be thrown away. I asked her to tell me which trash and I would go get her. She told me she couldn't tell me. I asked if she would sell it to me for $1.50? She did. Even though my heart was in so many pieces at the loss of my four babies, God was still telling me that in my brokenness I could praise Him.

The name of this figurine is Isabel. These days I reread and remind myself that even though my precious daughter Avery is on a difficult journey, we are still able to praise the Lord for the time he continues to give us with her. With my permission, if you would like to use this to encourage all the MBC ladies, please do. I send along a prayer that God will use this to touch the heart of all who read it and give them strength to praise Him in their pain and brokenness.

God bless you, Lynne (Avery Harrison's mom)

For Isabel

A broken-winged angel
still can sing
Sweet, sweet praises to the
newborn King

Over the rainbow and
beyond the stars

Is our sweet Lord and Savior
not the wizard of Oz!

God hangs tight with
broken winged angels
God's precious mercy will save
each fragile soul

A loving king - the Christ
who has risen
Touches each wounded heart
He died to make us whole.

Lynne Hendrix
1-21-1999

ANONYMOUS K's Journey

K was first diagnosed with breast cancer on April 1, 2014. She had felt the lump a few months prior but didn't think it was anything.

There is no history of breast cancer in her family and at the time she first felt the lump she didn't have insurance. When she got her insurance back she set up an appointment right away and was diagnosed from there. The diagnosis at that time was stage 2b ER/PR+ HER2-. She had a radical double mastectomy.

After pathology came back it turns out they did not get clear margins. The preliminary on her lymph nodes was wrong and there was cancer in them. She had to do six rounds of chemotherapy and three rounds of FEC followed by three rounds of Taxotere. She then had her exchange surgery and then she did six weeks of radiation. She was officially done with all treatment on New Year's Eve 2014.

Three weeks later she developed an infection in her right implant. It had to be removed and left out for five weeks so that the infection could heal properly and then it was replaced. She was put on Tamoxifen after that. However, it caused major issues with her menstrual cycle and she was bleeding so badly that her doctor called it 'flooding'. They did an ultrasound and found two masses on her ovaries. All of her doctors decided that it would be the best option for her to have a total hysterectomy. That was done and it turns out that the masses on her ovaries were pre-cancerous. She was put on a different hormone blocker for women in menopause called Exemestane.

She was on that when she was diagnosed Stage 4 in January 2019.

LYNNE HENDRIX

Mother of Avery Harrison whose Daughter says, "I Am Terminal!"

None of us walk through this journey alone. Even though at times we might think, 'How did we get to this point? Why did this happen to me?"

I am the mother of Avery Harrison. Avery was originally diagnosed with Stage IV Metastatic Breast Cancer HER2+ de novo to both breasts, hip, T2 of her spine and liver in 2014, at the age of thirty-eight. She did six rounds of chemotherapy plus Herceptin plus Pejeta, which seemed to work. Avery was declared No Evidence of Disease (NED) from the neck down. That is until the little buggers reared their ugly cancerous lesions and tumors again in 2016, at the age forty-one, when she received her second diagnosis of Stage IV Metastatic HER2+ Breast Cancer with Brain Metastasis. The past several years have seemed like a very bad dream. We are all ready to wake up from it.

Avery was raised to be very strong and independent, which has come in handy for this fight of her life. Although, at times, I can see in her eyes and hear in her voice that she is growing weary from this daily battle. Being an independent and determined young woman, it is difficult for her to let others help her with the simple daily life functions that so many of us take for granted. It has been hard on my heart to see my child become older than me over these seasons since her initial diagnosis.

My personality has always been one of being straight forward so that no one has to *read between the lines.* Avery has received some blunt and straight-forward talks from me in her life, but more so since her MBC diagnosis. Yes, I do have a very loving heart for my child; and yes, if I can encourage her to keep fighting, then I know why God put me here!

There are mornings/days when Avery and I speak and if she is having a bad day I ask, "How are you doing?" She blurts out "I AM TERMINAL!" Even though this is shocking to hear from your child the thing to remember is that we all are terminal. Some are running out of time a little faster than others. So cherish every single moment, enjoy every new sunrise, a reminder that you made it through the long night, every spectacular sunset, reminding you that you have made more memories, and do not ever pass up a time to wish upon a shooting star. Pray that a cure for MBC is right around the corner. Hug your loved ones and smile at that stranger who might look at you a little differently. Let them think that you know the secret of how to live. Most of all, give thanks to the One who made you and pray that God will give you a little bit longer time here on earth because we all are terminal.

My prayers are for all of you with MBC and your families. For such a time as this.

SANDRA GUNN No words

All words ring hollow after reading these expressions of fear of loss and unexpected Grief. There is no song in this breeze.

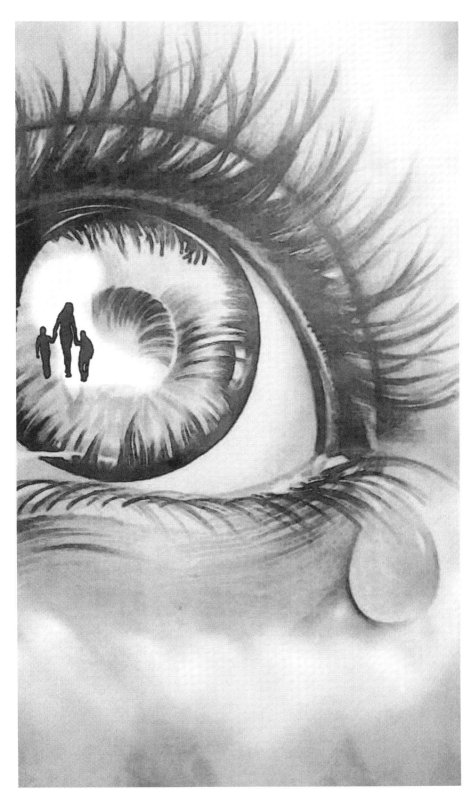

06. LAUREN HUFFMASTER
Be The Bridge

I WAS READING a thread on my favorite young adult cancer site and I ran across a friend who posted about how her heart is broken. Cancer treatments have left her infertile. It is a fact that most people outside of the cancer community don't think about. If your cancer is hormone driven, or you receive chemo, or radiation or many of the other treatments, your chances of having a healthy child after cancer are significantly diminished. I was fortunate enough to have three girls before my diagnosis, but many young adults are not so fortunate. Continuing on the thread, I read stories of other men and women who will never have the opportunity to be a parent and I was deeply saddened by their loss. Simultaneously, I became aware that as a stage four cancer patient, my three girls may one day find themselves without a mother.

So, on one end of the spectrum are a large number of young women unable to have children because of cancer and on the other, there are children who will one day be motherless because of cancer. These two groups of women need one another.

It is often through our tears that we discover hope. In our deepest hurt, the burden of our soul, there is an answer. In order to find the answer, though, we must open ourselves and our hurt to the world around us. One woman must be willing to embrace a child that is not her own while another must allow the kindness of a stranger enter her heart and her home. Both women must relinquish control of what they cannot control.

Life is much more about our weakness than our strength, yet we live as if the opposite were true. In weakness, we discover who we are. In weakness, we can share that true essence of our self. In weakness, we can truly experience kindness and love.

Strength, on the other hand, is nothing. Individual strength results in isolation.

Strength for the sake of independence or stature, personal satisfaction or bragging rights does not lead to the abundant life that is marketed in commercials. If you Google quotes about *strength* you find ancient wisdom passed down from every religion and region of the world. The quotes do not talk about financial success or physical stature. Instead, they speak of how one only finds strength when living in community, alongside others, bonded in weakness.

We have been sold a myth that strength is valuable above all else. Why else do we pretend that everything is ok? Why do we live in isolation, yearning for the closeness of a friend? Why is it nearly impossible to ask for help? Why do we work ourselves into anxiety attacks and heart attacks? Even when our body screams out for help, our mouth never admits a lacking of *strength.*

Strength is nothing but a lie, a lie that we have bought, and bought, and bought; but the greatest product of strength is isolation. Because of strength, each one of us sits on an island of isolation wishing for close friends and someone to help carry the load. The truth is, there is someone sitting in the house next door to you, wishing for the same thing. The person in front of you in line, the man in the cubicle across from yours, and the mom at the park are all sitting on their island of "strength" looking out at the isolation.

I would like to propose a change of perspective. Let's make weak the new strong. Weakness looks like a cancer survivor who cannot have children embracing a child and allowing love to flow forth from her wounds. Weakness looks like a mother with Stage 4 breast cancer welcoming a woman into the lives of her children so the children may experience love and acceptance from a new source. Weakness looks like two women looking into her own heart and seeing the greatest pain of her life, then using this brokenness to heal the brokenness in others, and perhaps, finding herself healed along the way.

Weakness looks like an act of kindness. Kindness is an unexpected, intentional investment in another individual with no thought of repayment. Kindness builds connection, the type that every person craves. Kindness is a cure for isolation, a bridge. Kindness eliminates individual strength. Kindness is a path toward strength, not individual strength, but instead a strength of purpose, a strength found in community, a strength with no thought of self. To give kindness requires the giving of time, or money, or emotion with no guarantee of personal gain. Kindness weakens the individual and this sacrifice of the individual results in a strengthening of community.

The role of strength and weakness is a paradox. Our constant pursuit of individual strength has, in fact, left us weak as individuals and as a community. Yet a willingness to embrace our own weaknesses enables us to be fortified by the kindness of others and able to build strong communities. It is in weakness that we can begin understanding the power kindness possesses.

Therefore, I urge us to contemplate the possibility that the pursuit of individual strength is not best, instead let us embrace the pursuit of kindness.

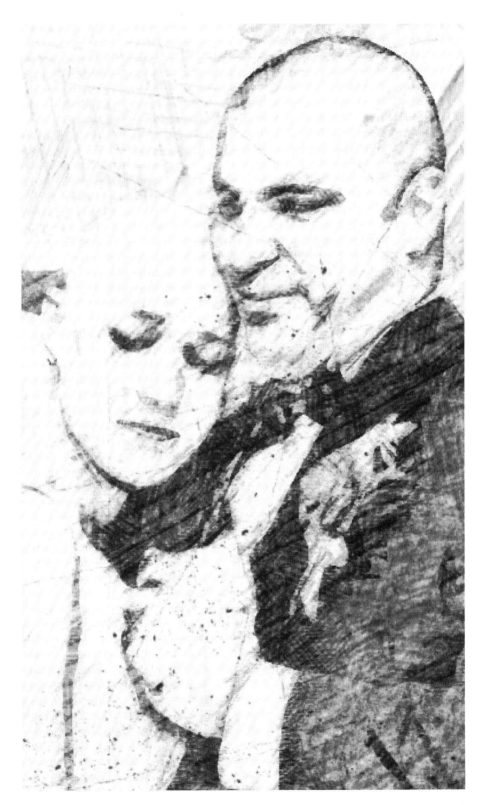

07. MICHAEL BANK
Death of a Queen

OBITUARY 10/21/18

Laurin Long Bank, COLUMBIA, SC - Died October 21st with her loving husband Michael Bank by her side. She was born to the late Dr. Gerald and Faye Long in Chapin, SC. Laurin was a graduate from W. Wyman King Academy in 2007. She continued her education at Midlands Technical College and graduated with an Associate of Arts in 2009 and then went on to earn a Bachelor's in History from USC Upstate in 2011. Later she went to Columbia College and received her Bachelor's in Business Concentration in Accounting in 2016. She had a love of life and her passions were traveling, adventures, and running. In addition to her husband, she is survived by her four brothers, Geoffrey, Russell, Richard, and David, and two sisters, Erin and Kristen and their spouses and their children with numerous aunts, uncles, and cousins. There will be a Celebration of Life Thursday, October 25th at the Tree of Life Congregation at 6719 N. Trenholm Road. Following the service, there will be a party! Instead of flowers the family's request donations to In The Middle or Leslie's Week.

October 22 at 7:02 AM
From Mike

It is with great sadness that we say goodbye to our beautiful queen. Yesterday morning she was feeling very weak and off, but still seemed to be doing fine. After getting her home from her aunt's house we could not get her comfortable. We had morphine brought in which didn't help.

She has left a huge hole in all of our hearts and I am humbled to be her king. I was able to carry her to bed and hold her until her last beautiful breath.

I know she has influenced so many people and she wants to be remembered as a celebration, not as a time for sadness. I will keep everyone updated on here as to arrangements. It's been my honor to be by her side the past three and a half years and I would not trade the memories that we have made for anything in the world. She has made me so much a better person.

Her humble king...
Mike

I do know for a fact she does not want any flowers and would rather have donations to https://www.facebook.com/inthemiddlebc/ or https://www.facebook.com/LesliesWeek/

Polka.dot.queen
October 22 at 4:35 PM
From: Mike

Laurin always hated the phrase that someone lost their battle with cancer... So, I asked her how she wanted to be described. It took her a couple weeks to come up with this answer.

And I do feel like this word 100% describes Our Queen.

I know I haven't responded to a lot of messages I've gotten, but please know I'm reading them and feel your love

Mike

For·ti·tude
/'fôrdə‚t(y)o͞od/
noun
courage in pain or adversity.

"she endured her illness with great fortitude"
synonyms: courage, bravery, strength of mind, strength of character, moral strength, toughness of spirit, firmness of purpose, strong-mindedness, resilience, backbone, spine, mettle, spirit, nerve, pluck, pluckiness, doughtiness, fearlessness, valor, intrepidity, stout-heartedness, endurance.

Polka.dot.queen
October 22 at 7:41 PM
From Mike

Per Laurin's wishes, we will have a celebration of life service. She wants it to be a joyful celebration in her memory.

Tree of Life Congregation
6719 N Trenholm Rd, Columbia, SC 29206
6:00 PM on Thursday the 25th

Polka.dot.queen
October 25 at 12:04 PM
From Mike

As we prepare for Laurin's celebration of life this afternoon. I have been reading messages from all around the world. I am so grateful to be so loved and have such a strong support system.

So, for today I decided to post our wedding video so that people can join us in celebration of our beautiful queen. She fought so hard to make it to our wedding day, March 24th, 2018, exactly 3 years from the day that we met. It was the perfect day in so many ways and not a dry eye in the room. So many people went above and beyond to make this our most precious memory.

The polka dot queen's humble husband…

Polka.dot.queen
October 26, 2018
From Mike

This is the final picture taken of our polka dot queen. This was taken Saturday evening in St Augustine Florida. Laurin was always the happiest and most relaxed by the beach and had an amazing last few days with her Aunt Vonnie being spoiled by her and her friends.

As difficult as this time is for me, my heart is in a good place. Laurin's biggest fear was a slow health decline and losing her quality of life. Up until only a few minutes before she passed, she was still having conversations with me, moving around and being her naturally crazy self. Although she was uncomfortable that day she maintained a phenomenal quality of life.

Her celebration of life service last night was very beautiful. In her wishes, she stated that we were only allowed to have ninety seconds of sadness, and then we were to have a party! Although Laurin was not Jewish, she wanted the same rabbi that married us seven months before to perform the service. Laurin always considered herself spiritual, as well as believed in a higher power, but did not follow a specific religion. She had been doing some counseling with the rabbi to process everything, and she had a huge amount of respect for him.The synagogue had standing room only last night and was so filled with love and joy. I appreciate everyone who came out to support me and her family. Her wishes were to be cremated and her ashes to be spread in the ocean. Today I have the difficult duty of picking up her remains. And tomorrow a few of her siblings and I are going out on a boat to fulfill her final wish.

Tomorrow morning, please keep Laurin on your mind as I say my final goodbye and return her to her favorite place.

Much love,
The polka dot queen's humble king…

Polka.dot.queen
October 27, 2018
From Mike

Laurin underwent the incredibly difficult task of preparing for her own departure. She was terrified to do it but wanted to relieve me of the burden. She wrote her own eulogy for the state paper, so if you read it these are her words, not mine.

She was planning on writing a final post for the blog as well but did not get to it. As I was going through her folder of important paperwork this quote was in there as well. So please take a moment this morning to read this and let the words sink in. It is so much the way Laurin thought and lived.

I'm Not Here

Don't stand by my grave and weep
for I'm not there, I do not sleep
I am a thousand winds that blow

I am the diamonds glint on snow
I am the sunlight on ripened grain
I am the gentle autumn's rain

When you awaken in morning's hush
I am the swift uplifting rush
Of quite birds in circle flight
I am the soft stars that shine at night
Do not stand at my grave and cry
I am not there, I did not die.

This morning Laurin's brothers and I are taking a boat out onto the Atlantic ocean to fulfill her final request of having her ashes scattered in the ocean. As we say our final goodbye, I want to remember all of the overwhelming love and support we have had from friends, family, and members of this page. So many people did so much to make our final year amazing. Thank you all, near and far, for the support. I plan on continuing this page in her legacy to teach others the lessons we discovered on how to truly live and love...

Much love,
The polka dot queen's humble king…

Polka.dot.queen
October 28, 2018
From Mike

Yesterday Laurin's brothers, one very close friend and I set out from Murrals inlet to scatter her ashes. On our way out, we were met by a pod of about twenty dolphins. We paused our journey to watch them play as they came within twenty feet of the boat.

We headed out to paradise reef off the coast since that sounds like somewhere Laurin would have chosen. We all spoke a few words and had a prayer and I took the honor of fulfilling her final wish.

Laurin was always happiest at the beach and her pain always seemed better managed by the ocean. As soon as she was released, the sun started shining through the clouds and it looked like there were millions of diamonds surrounding us on the water. The chop of the waves was about three feet so we had a wet ride coming back in. The pod of dolphins escorted us for about five minutes as we returned to the dock.

I spent the day wandering the beach, having wine and dinner by the ocean just like I would have if she was with me.

As much as she is missed, my heart is at peace knowing that I was able to give her more memories in three and a half years than most have in a lifetime. But my brain has no idea how to handle this and what to do next. I will be taking some time for soul-searching and figuring out what my next adventure is...

I'll keep everyone updated

Much love,
The polka dot queen's humble king...

Polka.dot.queen
October 29, 2018
From Mike

I was talking to one of my most trusted friends/mentor about this quote the other night. And I told him I can attest that it is 100% true. Laurin was a special person that few people are ever fortunate enough to meet in their life, much less fall in love with.

I have had so many friends come up to me and tell me how much they've seen me change and grow as a person since I met my lovely Queen. She taught me the meaning of unconditional love, made me not afraid to express my emotions, and learned to find so much more joy in this world.

I have always been an incredibly Mission focused person and thought that I didn't have time to deal with emotions. For those of you who don't know much about me, I'm the type of person who has always been on a strong mission. I've been martial arts for almost twenty-five years and hold the rank as one of the youngest martial arts Masters in the country. I run one of the most successful martial arts schools in the country, as well. I am an eagle scout as well as a highly decorated combat veteran. I competitively fought in martial arts tournaments, and wrestling matches for many years with very high levels of success.

I write this today not to brag on myself, but with all my experiences I thought I was prepared for almost everything until I met Laurin. Although I've accomplished so much, I never found true happiness until I learned to put my guard down and just start loving and living. The world can be a scary place, and for that, I felt highly prepared. But by focusing on that, I never noticed how loving the world can be, how many amazing and special people can be out there. It was like we should just live, love, and laugh every day.

As I've been thinking about how to carry-on Laurin's Legacy, I would like to use this page to share these lessons I've learned from her that have helped make my life so much more meaningful. As of right now, I don't know if I'm going to continue posting every day or occasionally. I would like you to keep your eyes on this page to help Inspire others to grow themselves, to be happier, and to live life on a higher level.

I look forward to being able to continue serving as Laurin did to help make the lives of everyone around us better.

Much love,
The polka dot queen's humble king…

Polka.dot.queen
October 30, 2018
From Mike

Every day since Laurin passed away I have been waking up at 4 AM. It did not matter if I went to bed at 10 PM or 2 AM. The last time I woke up this early was 2007 before I got out of the military. After a couple of days, I started getting very curious as to why I have been waking up this early.

Now that I have several extra hours in the day I have time to research. After some searching, I found that according to Chinese medicine this is the time of day where your energy is focused on your lung meridian. This is the time of day when your body processes grief and sadness that has not been dealt with internally.

As you can imagine, last week I had people with me 24/7 and several people staying at my house. But as of Sunday, everyone had gone home and it's just me and Smiley. I spent the day yesterday dealing with insurance, bank accounts, credit cards, and probate court. Afterward, I went to a fundraiser one of Laurin's good friends put on for In The Middle. We went out and had drinks afterward. A friend who is a massage therapist offered to give me a massage.

I was able to get far more done than I expected yesterday and am waiting on several callbacks today to finish things up.

I know I will keep finding more and more in the coming months but I am trying to finish as much as I can this week.

Today I have several friends who I am supposed to see and many more phone calls to make. I am hoping to spend the majority of the rest of the year traveling. For those who have known me for a long time don't be surprised if I reach out if I am in your area. Laurin wanted me to keep working on my bucket list adventures, 2 that I would really like to do before the end of the year are to drive a convertible along the entire California coast and see the northern lights.

No plans are made yet, but if you have any great ideas for me to do these please let me know.

Much love,
The polka dot queen's humble king

Polka.dot.queen
October 31, 2018
From Mike

Why did I decide to put up this video on Facebook? Because it was hilarious, it was fun, it was just like the rest of our relationship, all about having a good time together.

I was married once before I met Laurin. I actually ended up meeting Laurin a few weeks after I was legally separated. So needless to say, I was at a rough point in my life and Laurin had just finished her first round of chemo. Most of my friends told me it was too soon for me to get back out there, and Laurin's friends thought she was nuts for going out at that point in her life. On top of everything else, we met three weeks before she had her double mastectomy. And she was preparing to go to Durham NC for six weeks of radiation. With all of this, we just focused on trying to have fun while we were together. Which continued throughout our three and a half years together.

We both had every reason imaginable to not want to be in a relationship. So, we didn't focus on it. We decided on our first date as we sat on what we refer to as our, "shit bench," where we both discussed all the shit in our lives for an hour. We decided that we could each go through our own shit on our own, or we could try and go through it together. I immediately noticed her zest for life, and how she was unlike any woman I had ever met. I later found out she was pissed at me at the end of that date that I did not try to kiss her.

She was getting ready to move the next day so I did not see her, but we messaged back and forth all day. Then the next day before the Friday she was supposed to move, her sister, who was supposed to come with her large SUV, was unable to make it to help her. Laurin was going to try and completely move herself in her small Toyota Matrix. When she told me that my response was, "I have a truck period". After about thirty minutes of convincing, she finally allowed me to come over and our second date was moving. As soon as I got there, she pinned me against the wall and kissed me, I guess she wanted to set a good tone for the relationship.

Between my truck and her car, we were able to get pretty much everything in one trip. The next day she had some of her brothers coming to help her with the larger items. When reflecting back upon my first marriage I realize that I never really felt like I could be myself during my first marriage. For those who know me, know I have either a G-rated super corny sense of humor, or am completely inappropriate. There is pretty much no in-between. With Laurin, I felt comfortable just being myself on either end of the spectrum.

Please take the time you have to live laugh and love. Be yourself and do things that truly bring joy into your life. What Laurin and I had was so incredibly special. I learned so much about joy and living from her and wouldn't change the experience for anything in the world.

Over the past two days, I have been dealing with all of the legal parts of the estate - setting up probate, contacting banks, credit card companies, insurance companies etc. I think I have done about everything that I can. Everything else is a waiting game. I have to wait on the courts to open probate and the insurance companies to process the claims.

Keeping busy has been good, but now as things calm down I know that reality will start to sink in as I come home to a big empty house. Having a dog definitely helps, but I know a hole has been left in my heart that will never be filled. Fortunately, I have so many amazing friends around to help keep me busy, some days I know I will be very social - and some days I will need my time to process.

I appreciate all of the support from everyone on this Facebook page, and all the recommendations on possible things to do and places to go. As I finalize plans I will keep everyone updated.

The polka dot queen's humble king…

Polka.dot.queen
November 3, 2018
From Mike

That dreadful day…

Laurin's 2nd cancer Journey started on the same trip we got engaged. After having the most magical evening of our lives, June 13th, 2017, on an impromptu road trip to Niagara Falls and Laurin saying 'yes' to that magic question, we began the difficult leg of our journey.

On this 2000+ mile trip, Laurin started having back pain. She was starting a new job as soon as we got back, but originally figured it was from so much driving. The day before she was supposed to start working we ended up going to the ER for her back pain. They diagnosed it as severe muscle spasms and told Laurin to rest for two days. Over the next few weeks, the pain kept getting worse. There were several days she was so uncomfortable that she was afraid to drive home so I would have to pick her up. We started thinking she must have a bulging disk or something like that so we scheduled an appointment with an orthopedist. They sent her in for some scans and sent us home and told us they would contact us with the results.

This weekend was the weekend of the Eclipse last August. That weekend I had a scuba certification class scheduled, as well as a test for eight black belts going for advanced degrees. Saturday shortly after some good friends got into town we got a call from the orthopedist saying we needed to contact our oncologist ASAP! We proceeded to call the on-call oncologist and he recommended going ahead and admitting Laurin so they could start all the tests.

Unfortunately, they found the cancer was back. Sunday morning, after a sleepless night, I had to do my open water dive to finish my certification. All of Laurin's siblings were around, as they had a ton more tests for Laurin. I could not see her anyway. Then that afternoon, I had to run a test for the eight black belts going for advanced degrees, which is a grueling four-hour long test. I had not told any of them what was going on until after the test.

That night, I spent several hours with Laurin. They wanted to keep her in the hospital for a few more days. Some friends who came with us were there for the eclipse, so that Sunday I visited Laurin in the morning, came home to watch the eclipse, and then was back with Laurin the rest of the night.

Now things had calmed down and we had to face the reality of the situation. Laurin looked at me in tears asking me if I was still going to marry her. This crushed me to hear her ask that question. I assured her that I was 100% committed to marrying her and being by her side every step of the way. We had already started planning our wedding and the doctors encouraged us to move up the date.

We discussed all the possibilities and decided we wanted to stick with our chosen date, which was three years from the day we met. We were incredibly fortunate to have the nonprofit, In The Middle, offer to help us with the wedding, as well as a friend who used to be a wedding planner. We gave them everything we had and let them take over planning our wedding.

Meanwhile, we had to do the things most couples never think about. We met with an attorney for wills, power of attorney, and a prenup designed to help protect me in case of terrible medical bills. We did premarital counseling trying to plan a life, not just a marriage. We decided that we wanted to focus on quality over quantity in our lives. The thought of marrying someone that you are almost certain to lose within maybe months, maybe years if your lucky is terrifying. But I was committed to whatever time we had left, making it as special as it could be.

I have heard countless stories of husbands running after a diagnosis, and I refused to be a coward like that. Laurin had been such an amazing person and made me so happy, I was honored to be by her side every step of the journey.

Of course, if you have been a member of this blog for a while or read through the old posts, there have been many ups and downs, crazy adventures, and sleepless nights. I had the opportunity to write one of the most amazing love stories of all time and took to that task wholeheartedly. I have been a fighter all of my life and trained fighters for the past twenty years of my life. So it was my time to be Laurin's cornerman as she prepared for this journey.

I hope this helps fill in some of the gaps for those who have been following this journey, and I ask husbands and caregivers to make a decision today what you would do facing this information. Decide ahead of time the type of person that you will become. If you end up in my shoes, there is no hesitation. You will know exactly what to do...

Much love,
The polka dot queens humble king...

Polka.dot.queen
November 8, 2018
From Mike

Rant/Lesson here

Yesterday, I received a call from Laurin's life insurance company telling me that I was not listed as the beneficiary on her life policy. Now, I had no doubt that I was because I remembered scanning the documents for her to send in a few weeks before the wedding. I tried to talk to them and all they said was, "I'm sorry for your loss."

Fortunately, Laurin was very organized so I went through her paperwork and found the form rescanned it and sent it to them, to which they still replied that that did not matter because it was not on file with them. I was afraid I was about to go into a legal battle with an insurance company which is an uphill fight the entire way.

Fortunately, I remembered that I still have Laurin's phone which is logged into her email account. So I went through her sent messages from back before the wedding and found the email where she sent it to the insurance company, as well as the email where they confirm receipt of it.

After sending it to them, they gave a brief apology and said everything should be fine. I know a lot of couples keep all their information separate but if I did not have access to her account I would not have received this policy and the insurance company could have cared less. Hopefully, now everything will work out the way Laurin's wishes were. I wanted to share the story because if it happened to me I'm sure it could easily happen to lots of other people. Please make sure that your loved ones have access to your accounts and print out any confirmation emails and put it with your important paperwork.

Fortunately for me, we knew we had a short time left so we had many things in order which prevent me from having to make tough decisions when I was filled with grief. Please take some time today to make sure all your important documents are gathered. Take time to call the companies to make sure they have the policies updated especially if you've had any life-changing event recently. Because at the end of the day, the insurance companies don't even care about your wishes, all they care about is the paperwork in their system.

There are a few other insurance stories that I will tell as I'm at the point where I'm dealing with them, but you never know if you're going to get hit by a car today. Take a little bit of time every day to ensure those that you love most are taken care of.

Much love,
The polka dot queen's humble king…

Polka.dot.queen
November 21, 2018
From Mike

Happy polka dot Wednesday everyone!

For all of the new followers, polka dot Wednesday was created as a way to increase awareness of Stage 4 cancer in honor of our Polka Dot Queen. Every Wednesday, Laurin's feed has been filled with people tagging her in pictures of them wearing polka dots! It always made her day and helped her feel loved!

I am back home from my DC/NY trip, and I am heading to the beach tonight for Thanksgiving with some friends. I do appreciate the massive number of people who have reached out to make sure I have somewhere to go for Thanksgiving. I am still trying to decide what direction I want to focus on next in my life, but so far taking time for myself has been very therapeutic. It was definitely very tough to come back to an empty home, and I still have so much to do. But one day at a time, I'll slowly get the house back in order and continue to get Laurins affairs in order.

I am still waiting on the state to officially open probate, but collection calls are already coming in. Fortunately, they don't have my number, so I just see it on Laurin's phone, and I am already getting letters in the mail. But there is nothing I can legally do until probate is opened. I'm sure the next few weeks will be difficult as I decide what to do with everything, but I would rather deal with it sooner than later.

Everyone enjoy your Thanksgiving and never take this family time for granted.

Much love,
The polka dot queen's humble king…

Polka.dot.queen
December 21, 2018
From Mike

Today marks 2 months since I lost my queen. I do feel blessed with all if the overwhelming support from all my friends. All the travel has been good for my soul.

Fortunately, I was able to get the convertible sold this week, thanks to one of my good friends who works at a dealership. Fortunately, there should only be a few minor parts of her estate to finalize when I get back. I still have to go through her office and a few other little things to get the house back in order, and then figure out final tax returns for her.

Otherwise, when I get back, I know its time to get going on my new normal. Time to get back training in martial arts, time to catch up with friends, time to get my next set of goals moving forward at work, time to design what I want my life to look like in the coming years. Time to plan more bucket list adventures!

I have always been an avid goal setter, which I have put on the back burner as the only goal that mattered to me was taking the best possible care of Laurin.

I have no doubt that I will still think of her daily, and always remember the amazing adventures we had together. But we also had the tough conversations, and I know that she wants great things for me. Every step will be difficult, but she has definitely taught me that we only live once and there is no excuse to not live it to the fullest.

When Laurin was rediagnosed, we had a long conversation about wanting to make sure that when her time came that I would not be left wishing and wondering if I could have done more. We lived in such a way that I can proudly say that I don't wish I could have done anything differently. We lived on our terms.

Now as the holiday weekend is coming, up let's all spend some time not just making resolutions but designing the life that we truly want. This is not easy and takes lots of time. But if Laurin taught us all anything, it is how to live. For those that are closest to me and will probably get sick of me talking about this, but I want to see everyone around me bring their lives to the next level as well.

I'll keep everyone updated on my public goals, and I hope to keep inspiring brothers and others!

Much love,
The polka dot queen's humble king

January 8, 2019
From Sandra Gunn

Dear Humble King,

You have inspired all the men in our LESLIE'S WEEK families. Your positive outlook is comforting to many who are grieving the loss of their Stage 4 Breast Cancer wives. Your journey, which is filled with good advice and Laurin's laughter in the midst your grief, leaves a mark in the Universe of Love.

I Heard Your Voice in The Wind Today
Suzannah Richards, by permission

I heard your voice in the wind today
And I turned to see your face;
The warmth of the wind caressed me
As I stood silently in place.

I felt your touch in the sun today
As its warmth filled the sky;
I closed my eyes for your embrace
And my spirit soared high.

I saw your eyes in the window pane
As I watched the falling rain;
It seemed as each raindrop fell
It quietly said your name.

I held you close in my heart today
It made me feel complete;
You may have died but you are not gone
You will always be a part of me.

As long as the sun shines…
The wind blows…
The rain falls…
You will live on inside of me forever
For that is all my heart knows.

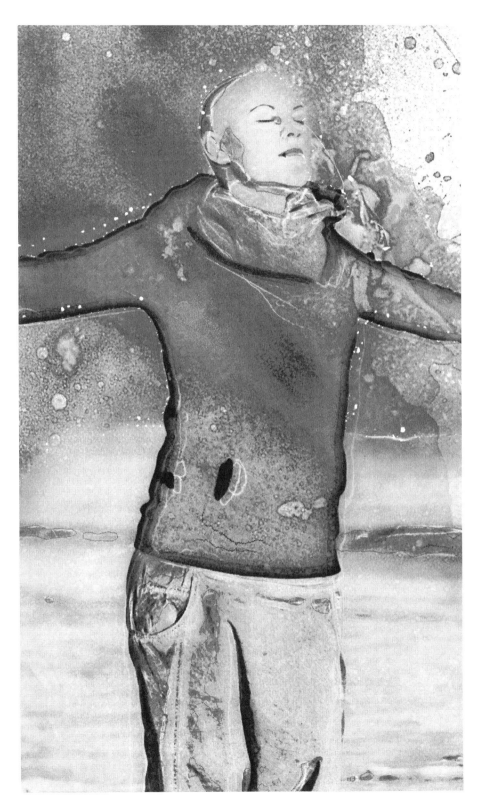

08. LAUREN HUFFMASTER
A Gift of Cancer!

CANCER TREATMENTS create a massive physical struggle and a daily fight for survival. Constant medical scrutiny leads to insecurity. Treatments strip and take away strength, both physical and mental. Then one day, my last treatment is done and it hits me: What comes next? Is the cancer gone? How will I know? Isn't there anything else that can be done? Where do I go from here? The season after treatment is very difficult, filled with emotional instability, questions, fear, and uncertainty.

Unfortunately, for many of us, once treatments are complete, we enter a season of feeling stuck in post-treatment anxiety. There are many fears and unanswered questions. These thoughts fill us with a new type of need. They are needs that cannot be easily revealed nor clearly communicated. How do I start again? Has everyone already forgotten that I had cancer? How will I pay for these past two years? How long before this all begins again? What is this pain in my side? On and on the questions roll, controlling our emotions and crushing our ability to thrive.

In this emotional process of beginning again, the question, "Who am I?", emerges. This question might seem trite, but in this season of significant change, it deserves proper attention before we are able to heal emotionally.

Before cancer, I would have described myself as a confident, centered person on the best path for my life. Then my life stopped. I was stripped of my confidence and my path. I was left with nothing but the question, "Who am I?". All of the adjectives I would have used to answer the question before cancer, no longer apply. At the same time, I came face to face with new truths about myself. Before cancer I would have stated with confidence, "I am more than my circumstances", yet when terrible circumstances came my way, I was left changed and shaken. Before cancer I would never have thought, "I am defined by my physical appearance", yet when my hair fell out with my eyebrows and eyelashes, I truly struggled to find myself in the mirror and other places.

Cancer's impact on my self-image showed me that I have a lot of room for growth. The truth is that I am more complex than I will ever know. There are pieces of myself that I put on and bring forward daily for all to see. There are parts I do not even want to show myself. Upon honest examination, there is an unknown number of layers that make up who I am. Each significant story in my life created a layer. Some layers happen to fall on the surface and receive the spotlight while others lay hidden despite their significant value.

One exercise for escaping post-treatment anxiety, is to take time to find an honest answer to the question, "Who was I?", and the follow-up question, "Who do I want to be?". These are not easy questions to resolve. I am fractured. I am different at work than at home. My ideal 'me' is different from who I am every day. There are many versions and many visions of myself. Fortunately, this complexity provides an opportunity for who I can become.

Cancer took at least one version of me. It disappeared and was left in my past. As treatments end, it is important for me to take time to mourn for that version of me. I have spoken with survivors who wrestle with picking up the pieces in order to put that old 'self' back together with minimal success. I feel we must be reminded that whatever picture of self that was lost during cancer is not the only version of you. Perhaps it is not even the best version of you.

Cancer stripped me of both good and bad, but I have the ability to rebuild. I have the power to recreate myself not as who I was, but who I want to be. I have the opportunity to minimize the negative aspects of my life and replace them with how I want to define my future.

Post-treatment is a unique moment of time to become whomever I want to be. It is a moment of vulnerability and rawness. A moment when I am not healed but I have moved beyond the sickness. There is stillness, as the routines of life have not swept in, but there is also churning within my thoughts. My old expectations are gone along with many of my fears. So, what do I want for myself now? Post-treatment is a season of freedom. Freedom is a gift that is both liberating and terrifying, and beginning again requires significant courage.

Let us fortify ourselves as we consider who we are.

As cancer survivors, we have accomplished an impossible task. There was something in our life, in our body, trying to kill us. We made difficult decisions, that only we could make. Perhaps when we received the diagnosis, there was no question that we would proceed with treatment, or perhaps we struggled with where to begin. Either way, it requires significant courage to willingly submit oneself to chemotherapy, radiation, and surgery.

Once treatment begins, it requires more and more courage to continue through the process. The night before a scheduled chemo is filled with choices. Can I handle another treatment? Do I want what tomorrow will bring? Then despite the knowledge of what is to come, we move forward, pushing through treatments and in the end accomplishing impossible things. We pushed back a disease that wanted to kill us. We beat the odds. We are triumphant. We are fierce. We are strong. We may not feel it today, but it is there inside of us. If we choose to own this piece of our new self it can monumentally change how we answer, "Who do I want to be?"

I am choosing to embrace the strengths cancer revealed and I have placed this strength on the surface of my new identity. I consider this a gift of cancer. Before cancer, I would never have described myself as fierce, but now, if I am honest, I know that inside of me is a strength that will rise against any challenge in my life. I can face any impossibility with confidence. I have done impossible things, I can do it again. I have pushed through crippling fear, I can do it again. I have submitted all that I am in order to accomplish a goal, I can do it again. I am driven by a deep unshakable confidence and courage that I never experienced before cancer. As I learn to walk in this new strength, I become more and more thankful for my cancer experience.

So, who am I? I was changed by cancer that is true, but how I was changed plays an important role in my future. The presence of cancer in my life did not change me, there were months or possibly years when I had cancer in my body and I was unaware. My life began to change because of what I chose to believe about myself and others after I heard the words, "You have breast cancer." Through treatments, did I believe I was all alone in my fight or that I was surrounded by a community? As a survivor do I believe I have overcome cancer, or do I only have a few years before the fight begins again? It is what I choose to believe that changes me, not the cancer itself.

Cancer provides a platform for deep reflection. It showed me what was already inside of me. It revealed my insecurities and fears. I cannot blame cancer for the baggage that was already present in my life, just as I cannot blame cancer for who I am. Cancer taught me many things and helped me take an honest look into the layers of who I am.

Now, what I choose to place on the surface, for all to see, is different than before. Now the characteristics I simply did not acknowledge before, I choose to embrace.

Who I am after cancer is not a puzzle needing to be put together in the correct way, but rather is one layer upon the next. Like the layers of the Earth, each layer tells a story. Each story cannot stand alone for they are all interconnected and require each other for a true understanding of all that I am. My cancer experience has become a layer in my life. A layer that tells a new story of who I am. Cancer is only one layer though, what I do with that part of my story, is up to me.

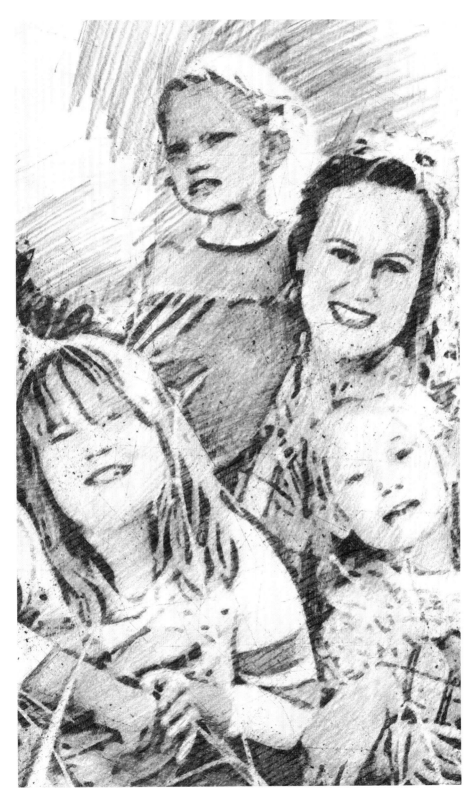

09. LETTERS TO
My Children

SANDRA GUNN 3/21/2019

I WAS IN RECOVERY from my first breast cancer mastectomy on April 4, 2013. I began to drift into a zone between heaven and earth as my thoughts became focused on my sons. If the worst were revealed to me what would I tell my sons? How would I let them know who I was and how I loved them? What life lessons would I communicate? How would I say in words their mother's vision for them?

I did not know where to begin or what words to use that would leave them with the essence of me and the love we shared throughout their lives. There were no words; there were only heartfelt emotional feelings that seemed inexpressible. At the time, I thought this would be an impossible task to write "Letters to My Sons". It was! I never wrote those letters, not because I did not want to, but because I could not find the words to say *goodbye*.

I asked our Book Collaborators Club to contribute to this chapter. Three responded many said they would. But like me, they could not find the words that equaled the emotions.

LAUREN HUFFMASTER 12/26/2018

With snow on Christmas Eve and the entire family all around, you can pretty much wrap it up to the best Christmas of all times. We are in beautiful Tahoe. We just had family pictures taken, and I got chilled to the bone. So then — all four of us jumped into the hot tub to warm up. While we were in the hot tub we sat and watched the sunset over the lake.

As I sit snuggled down in blankets, I look out over the vistas and watch as the tiny sliver of golden light silhouettes the amphitheater of mountains. With this beauty all around us, my mind turns to you - my three shining lights. The girls whose love keeps me warm. The girls who are my sunshine. The girls who bring me comfort, simply by being near. Without you, no view and no Christmas would ever be complete.

I think you are just getting old enough that I can sit and watch you. I observe how beautiful each of you are on the outside and how confident you are in your abilities. I sit without thinking and take in all that you are. I am reminded of when you were born. After I delivered each of you everyone wanted to hold you right away. They would take you away from me and marvel at your perfect little face. While you were put on display, my body would tense up and shake as if I was in the Arctic. Then as soon as you were handed back to me, I would relax, mind, body, and soul. My body stopped shaking and I would just stare into your little face.

As you grow, you pull away and spend time with others. Though this is normal, I think my body tenses again, like it recognizes the sensation of being separated from you. Here in Tahoe, on Christmas, I have not needed to cook and clean. Others have carried the responsibility of running the house and I have had the opportunity to sit, watch, and learn. I can look into your beautifulness and take you in. Take you in. It seems to be the right phrase for what it feels like.

So, as I take you in, I want to reflect for a moment. I have only good expectations for next year. My meds are working, my articles are written and the Foundation is founded. There seems to be nothing but promising endings on the horizon. But in case this year isn't filled with good things, I want to pause and write you a Christmas letter to say things that need to be said.

First, I want you to know that I have tried to be very honest with you about my cancer. I have given you the chance to ask questions and I have always answered honestly. Also, the parts you don't understand, I have done my best to explain in such a way that you can at least have an idea. The one thing I have not done is look you in the eyes and tell you that stage 4 cancer leads to death. There is no cure.

Let me tell you why I haven't done this. First, you are little girls! You were two, four, and six when I was diagnosed. I want you to walk in confidence rather than finding yourself burdened by something that is too difficult for most adults to carry. Secondly, I am full of hope. If you read through my writings, I declared to the world my unquestionable belief that I will not die from cancer. But if I have misunderstood God's purposes in my life, I want to write this down so that I may be understood. Then as you grow into true adults, you may see who I am on the inside and not struggle with questions about who I was.

I want you to know, I am not angry. I know I get frustrated with you when Daddy is gone for long periods of time, but I am not angry with you or God or Daddy or anyone. I am tired, exhausted actually. Emotionally and often physically as well, I am tired. I am often sad. I think I am mostly sad because I am tired. Feeling happy and fun for you is very hard for me. It requires that I let go of all the hurt and feel the freedom of joy for a moment. This part is good. Joy, silliness, pleasure, of course, all of that is good. The problem is that when that fleeting moment passes the sadness is so much stronger. So I don't often leave my numb-not happy, not sad space.

This hurts me because before cancer, before you can remember, I was the fun mom, the fun aunt, I didn't care if I was silly in public or at home. I was even driven to silliness because of my love for you. Right now, at least, all of that is gone. I just can't. I want more than anything, that you will forgive me. I don't want you to lose sight of your childhood too soon and I know that almost every day I steal a piece of it away.

I am thankful that Daddy is plenty silly. When he comes home, your hyper joy is not something that hurts but instead is an outlet that Daddy can facilitate with stories and wrestling matches and anything else you ask of him. He is a good Daddy and he recognizes my brokenness and is willing to be made a fool because of his love for you.

I want you to know that I push you to be strong independent girls. Everyone is baffled at the risks you are willing to take and adventures you face. Even when you don't feel strong, you are out there, traveling, hiking, climbing, skiing, singing, and so much more. This was all intentional. I wanted to thrust you into the lives of others, and not feel dependent on me.

This probably sounds like a terrible idea so let me explain my logic, for good or bad. Girls are typically pretty attached to their mom. Rightfully so, but it isn't really until the teenage years that youth find a new source of stability and affirmation in other kids. Other kids are not going to know how to support you when your mom is sick or even dies. So I have been very intentional to surround you with communities. You have the Huffmaster clan, Lili and Mimi and Duke. You know what it feels like for Mom and Dad to go away, even on extended stays. You have Camp Kesem and the support groups that come from them. You have your little school where everyone knows us and our story, and church, and more. I don't know who you will want to turn to if I get sick again, but I have given you options. You are strong enough to stand on your own. You are. You stand on stage and climb mountains. I know you can do this too! I believe in you and I am proud of you already.

I do want to give you a word of caution. If I get sick, it does not mean you have to grow up in that moment. It will feel like you do but fight the impulse! Daddy will find people who make you laugh and take care of everything you need. It won't be the same (of course not!) but it also does not make you the adult who must care for the family. It doesn't. Daddy will need some time. He has to adjust to becoming the only parent. It is going to be hard and he is totally going to mess up, (Sorry, hon, but you will.) So be patient. Forgive him. Love him even if nothing is going right. He needs you just like you need him. Don't let your anger or frustration over little things create more hurt for him or one another. Remember, Love is strong. It is the strongest, in fact. So if nothing is going right, just settle your heart and choose love. Make good choices.

Today I watched you, all dressed up for pictures. You are all so different. Audrey is a ray of love to all she meets, Hope is wild and free, and Sissa is soft and comforting. God made you each like this on purpose. Don't let any hurt change you. Hurt can change us if we choose to start down a dark path and sometimes it takes half a lifetime to come back out of it. Please don't let your disappointment in me, my words, my sickness, whatever - don't let it steal who you are. You are my legacy. I want you to live lives that honor me and Daddy. Sadness can come for the night but please LET joy come in the morning (Psalm 30:5). I don't want you to fake being happy but I don't want you to choose isolation or sadness. If you can find a choice, turn to the Light, and let God lead you toward His light. He understands what it feels like to lose your one and only mom, He lost His only son. He knows.

In my sickness, no one has been able to hear my hurt and my burden and not feel overwhelmed by my brokenness. For the past three years, God was my only outlet. I could not talk to friends really and couldn't dump my thoughts on Daddy because he had his own burdens and didn't need mine too. Daddy knows this. He trusts me and God and our relationship. Daddy knows that I will hear what I need to hear when I need to hear it. I had truly dark weeks and there are times I cried where no one could see me, but God always pulled me out. Even if my heart was breaking, I kept my heart turned toward God. I did not have the strength to reach out to Him, but I never turned my face from Him. I waited, watched, and hoped that He, who is my salvation, may save me. He never failed me. There may have been weeks when I had nothing but silence, but then God spoke - in the quiet stillness.

Girls, I have tried to teach you all I know about God. I lecture you on the way to school almost every morning. I am sure it feels like lectures but in reality, I am revealing my truest heart, my greatest treasure and I hope that you will receive it.

Knowing God is not a hard thing to do. It is only the position of the heart. You cannot work hard enough to hear Him. You cannot be kind enough to receive Him. You must sit, quietly, waiting just longer than you think is possible. Then when you hear even the simplest word, it changes everything. Relationship doesn't stop at hearing. Everyone thinks hearing is the difficult part. The hardest thing comes later, it is believing. What God speaks to you, you must trust more than any other thing in your life.

Yes, pray about it! Yes, wait and make sure your heart feels like it is continuing to open, rather than the opposite. But after you have tested it, TRUST IT. No one on this earth knows what God has in store for you. BUT I BELIEVE it is something big. My cancer story can push you into greatness or it can pull you into darkness. Please, listen to your heart. Figure out what it sounds like when you hear a lie (that you want to believe!) and then what it sounds like when something completely new emerges inside of you, even if it is hard to believe. Lies are easy to believe. They say, "no one understands me," "no one loves me," "God has forgotten me." If you hear such lies, don't worry! The deceiver told Jesus the same thing. Jesus knew the sound of the Father's voice and turned away from these lies, and you can too.

I encourage you to do a journal. Journal your prayers, He will answer them, and you can look back and see His presence in your life. You can write your questions and He will enlighten your mind to answers you never considered. Write, read, talk, and learn so that you may know what it feels like to walk through life with God. It is not something I can give you. I can point you in the right direction but I cannot open your heart in the right way. You must choose to do so.

Girls, forgive yourself for every time you talked back to me. Forgive yourself for not cleaning your room or fussing when asked to pick up dog poop. I have forgiven you. My love is bigger than these little hurts. Please receive this and know it to be true. Your mind will race, possibly for years to come, of all the things you could have done differently. Don't live in the past. It is done, it is finished. I release you from those disappointments. You were learning and growing and it was my job to teach you. That is all.

Find your purpose in this hurt. We are all going to be broken one way or another. For you, I am your first big pain. But I trust that you were given this as an opportunity. NO ONE expects you to rise above this easily. Just rise above it, so that your story, your testimony won't be lost. I have invested every day in YOU. You are my treasure, you hold more of me than anyone else on earth. I have loved you with all of my heart, all of my mind, all of my soul, and all of my strength. (Mark 12:30)

It was my duty and my joy. Please love one another as I have loved you.

I did not serve you that you may have an easy life. I served you that you may see what it looks like to be a servant. I am not perfect but please learn from me, serve one another, serve with a joyful heart. The act of serving is not a burden, it is a privilege. This is a great mystery that I don't expect you to understand but hold it in your heart until the day comes when you do understand.

ERICIA LEONARD 1/15/2019

Words to my children:

Where to begin? I have been trying to do this since day one and here we all are almost four years later and I am still not able to process these thoughts without a complete painful experience/meltdown.

I often cry because I feel that I have let you down as a mother. Parents are supposed to take care of their children, nurturing their dreams and aspirations while teaching them about life, showing them how to manage their own lifestyles and make positive decisions. In the natural order, we take care of you. And if needed, when we have aged, you take care of us. That all changed when I was diagnosed with Stage 4 breast cancer in July 2016.

It seems that from the start, I had the worst of luck. It seems that way because we have had many different issues, every setback, every hospitalization, every infection, every birthday missed. Trust me when I tell you I have talked to other survivors or Metastatic fighters, and it could be AND is worse for some.

Some women are all alone. Their families and friends have abandoned them. Some women are so young that they never had a chance to be on their own, get married, or have their own children. There are so many different stories and situations that I have talked about or read about with other women who have this horrible disease. It can and does take on so many catastrophic forms, and when that happens I always think of you three. I have you. I will always have you. You have and continue to be there for me. When my heart is breaking, I can count on my three beautiful daughters to make me smile. I can count on you to continue to love me through this.

You three are my rocks. I draw my daily, sometimes hourly, strength from you and your father. Without my family, my children in my life, I would NOT be able to go on. I want you to know this, try to understand why I fight so hard. Yes, it's for me but in reality, I'm fighting for you. I will never stop fighting for you. NEVER.

You are so young. You three have had to deal with all of this at such a young age, such an emotional, confusing, hard age. Being a young child and a teenager is hard enough without having to worry about your mom or her struggles. Let's be real here, MY struggles have had a direct impact on you. They have become YOUR struggles, your worry. Your sense of "normal" shattered the day when mine did, AND that's when I start to feel bad as a mom. Feeling like I haven't protected you or have been unable to shield you from this constant conflict and painful unknown. You have been there the whole time. It's frustrating. It's painful and heartbreaking.

One thing I want to make sure I tell you is *thank you.*

Victoria, Taylor, and Remington! Thank you! Thank you for taking care of me when I needed it; thank you for making me laugh when I needed it; thank you for all the hugs, kisses, smiles and constantly loving me when I needed it. Thank you for ALL your patience with me, thank you for all your sacrifices for me. Thank you for loving me through this.

Know that I want you to know I am always here. My love will NEVER stop.

Always and forever,

Mom

TINA ARGO 6/5/2019

To my son Cason,

Live life to the fullest and keep your family close always. Take God in your heart and keep him there. He will get you through all you endure. Follow all your dreams; do not let anyone stop you. I am so proud of you, and you have kept me fighting to go on. There will be hardships and struggles, but I know just like me, you will do fine. Keep your faith; You will shine like a rockstar !!!!!!! This life is what you make it, even when it throws hard balls to you, our motto is get up and fight till the end. Just know your mom is grateful and honored to call you my son, there isn't a day go by that I don't think of you. Even when God calls me home, I will be waiting for you to come there. Also, I love you son with all I have.

Love, your mom Tina

To my grandson Pace,

As you get older, please let God in your heart and allow Him to take care of you, my sweet little guy, You live your life to the fullest, happiness is what you will go for. I am so proud of you; you make this Nina happy in her heart; we always have laughs and great times with you. Memories, keep them in your heart to cherish. I want you always to remember to keep your family close, never turn your back on them sweet one, you have some great folks in your life, so glad of that. You are a fighter like your Nina, so I know you will do fine in life. I know you will make me proud. I have my eyes on you even if I am in another place. I will always be watching over you. I love you with all my heart, Pace.

Love, your Nina(Tina)

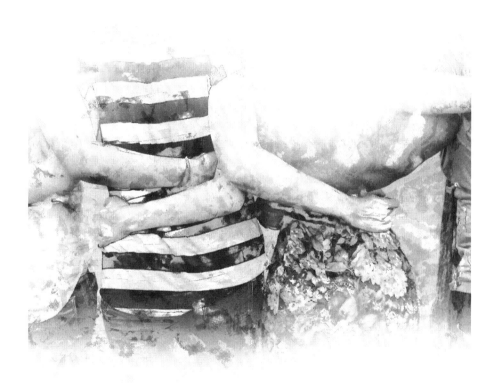

10. A TRIBUTE TO
Stage 4 Breast Cancer Women

WHO ARE THEY these Stage 4 Breast Cancer women who live on the edge of the breast cancer community? Who are they? How do they endure the assault on their bodies, minds, and self-esteem? How do they do this? What are their fears and how do they conquer them?

I ask, "Who are they?" They are women who know they are dying. They know there is no cure. Yet they go to bed and wake up each morning believing in life. They refuse to accept their diagnosis and prognosis. They believe they will make it. They live each day, every moment, in a light that only they can see. They care for their children, sometimes hold down the needed job, and comfort their husbands, if they are lucky enough to have one who does not abandon them. They know each touch, each feeling, each extension of themselves will leave a memory in their family aura. They live on a level of awareness that few women achieve who are not "survivors". They see through silliness, superficial personas, and shallow gestures. Their life is precious with not a moment to waste. Their time is relevant. Their goals are gently measured. Their treasures are human. And, I have found they appreciate the kindness of others beyond the ordinary. Kindness is a quality they treasure. It is a rarity, like a precious gem. Who are they? They are extraordinary.

How do they endure the assault on their bodies, minds, and self-esteem? In one of our GLAM4STAGE4 events, a Stage 4 Metastatic Breast Cancer woman was about to get her hair washed. She sat in the chair, looked at me, and broke down sobbing. I put my arm around her and asked, "Ineia, what is causing your tears on this joyful Day of Beauty?"

She responded, "Sandra, I am so ugly and my son gets married in two weeks. How can I go to his wedding looking like this?"

I told her, "You will not be ugly when you leave here today. You will be beautiful. You will be restored. Now, sit back and let Jamie do her job so she can begin your new look."

I turned at that moment to look in the room. It was frozen. Every technician was stunned. Some had tears. They became determined and began to comprehend their importance in the lives of the twelve women we were hosting. I watched as Ineia went from the wash-bowl and then to the chair to have her hair styled. The technician was totally infused with the grief and sorrow of her client, Ineia. An hour later her hair was complete. She stood and came over to me crying.

"Look at me Sandra! I am beautiful!" We cried as we hugged.

I held her and whispered, "You are the most beautiful mother your son will ever have."

She came back two weeks later to have her hair styled believing this is what made her beautiful. Ineia has an inner light that most are missing. Her beauty pours through her eyes and splashes over the person with whom she is engaged in conversation.

Why do they feel *ugly*? Is it because everything that society defines as beautiful in a woman is removed from them? They lose their breasts to mastectomies. They lose their hair to chemotherapy. They lose their skin texture to radiation; it is no longer soft and smooth but burned, cracked and peeling. They bear up under the most severe pharmaceutical onslaught in the clinical trials they volunteer to endure in the hope of finding a cure. They endure pharmaceutical side effects that would destroy a *normal* woman.

There are husbands who abandon them. They cannot look at them in their disfigurement. These men are doomed. They will never find happiness as they look for in physical beauty when it is only found in devout places they have never been. Their Stage 4 Breast Cancer wives know of these devout places. It is where they live every day. They are transformed by this disease. They find faith and it comforts them. It makes them whole. It gives them life that is beyond what mere mortals live. Stage 4 Breast Cancer women live with one foot on earth and the other in a spiritual world. They see beyond the physical. And, when they leave they are quiet, at peace, and filled with love. I have been with several and I see their departure. It is never noisy. It is near melodic.

Someone told me once, "There are no atheists in fox holes!"

What are their fears? When I asked this question they responded, "What will become of my children when I am gone? Who will love them as I do?" No one will love their children as they do and they know it. Hence, they become engaged with their children on levels that other mothers miss in their families. Stage 4 Breast Cancer women know the urgency of love, kindness, compassion, teaching, healing, and family strength. This is where they live. Every experience matters in a deeply profound way that is not easily expressed in words.

Stage 4 Breast Cancer women are not Heroes. They are not Warriors. They are not Fighting the Good Fight. They are coping in a world that few understand. They are living on an intuitive level that few understand. They internalize their fear to help their families from having fear. They hide their thoughts and manufacture those that make others comfortable. They live a reality that only they are able to cope with in order to protect their families from the emotional destruction that dwells within Stage 4 Breast Cancer. They are not Warriors. They are Angels Unaware.

This last chapter is my humble tribute to Them.

Ineia, Lauren Huffmaster, Tina Argo, Denise Hayes, Teresa Teaford, Ericia Leonard, Danielle Warren, Jeanette Rhile, Avery Harrison, Keeli Avars, Lisa Cooper Quinn, Shelby Quinley, Wendy Marie Nowicki, Nancy MacGillivray, Nina Lukenich, Michelle Hedman, Joy Ward, Emily Williams, Victoria Putnam, Ann Corinne Whitney, Georgiana Vernon, Angela Ratterman, Sara Zimov Levinson, Ivey Cline, Rhonda Howell, Cassie Newman, Amanda Holbrook, Sara Balaker, Kelly Prescott, Michele Mo, April Brown, Melissa Burke, Nicolette Ricci-Swabby, Dyanne Barnes, Joanne Mansfield, Karen Dean Byrne, Nina Mueller, Donna Watkins, Mary Ann Petrone, Maribel Rincon, Karen Jacobowitz, Heather Tewell-Youngs, Laurin Long Banks, Kim Dawn Kerns, Laura Williams, Melissa Ziemian, Lynn Hutchinson, Heather Harris Winkler, Jena Harmon, Renee Mundell, Losa Todd, Courtney Lasater, Marie Hutchins, Anita Wetter, Jennifer Hund, DeAnna Chase Raymond, and all of those Stage 4 Breast Cancer women across this great nation and the entire world.

...to all the Angels Unaware.

ABOUT THE AUTHORS

"If you want to go quickly, go alone. If you want to go far, go together"

I thank each of the 43 individuals who wrote this book with me. These are their words, their dreams, their sorrows, their joys, their emotions, their pain, and their last wishes to every woman who is diagnosed and lives with Stage 4 Metastatic Breast Cancer for the remainder of their lives.

THE STAGE 4 BREAST CANCER WOMEN	THE HUSBANDS
Tina Argo	Curtis Argo
Keeli Ayars	Ryan Ayars
Karen Byrne, DIED MAY 10, 2018	
Denise Hayes	
Amanda Holbrook	
Rhonda Howell	
Lauren Huffmaster	Clifton Huffmaster
Ericia Leonard	
Sarah Levinson	Joshua Levinson
Nina Muller, DIED DECEMBER 18, 2018	
Wendy Marie Nowicki, DIED APRIL 23, 2019	
Shelby Quinley	Brian Quinley
Lisa Cooper Quinn	
DeAnna Raymond, DIED MARCH 14, 2019	Shawn Raymond
Jeanette Rhile	
Teresa Teaford	
Danielle Warren	
Melissa Ziemian, DIED DECEMBER 25, 2018	Michael Ziemian

FAMILY MEMBERS

Anonymous..K's Journey
Linda Brand...Mother-In-Law of Danielle Warren
Jayme Ferris...Sister of Danielle Warren
Gigi...Mother of DeAnna Raymond
Sandra Gunn...Editorial Supervision and Author
Lynne Hendrix...Mother of Avery Harrison
Cason Jones..Son 15 Years Old
Taylor Leonard... 15 Years Old
Victoria Leonard.. Daughter 16 Years Old
PJ Morgan...Mother of Kelly Prescott
Jill Murray...Sister of Karen Byrne Dean
Delaney Rhile.. 9 Years Old, Poem to Mom
Kelly Snethen.. Mother of Danielle Warren
Michele Thompson.......................................Mother of Lauren Huffmaster

OTHER HUSBANDS

Michael Bank, WIFE DIED OCTOBER 21, 2018
Ryan Cassidy
Thomas Newman Jr.
Scott Petrone, WIFE DIED OCTOBER 27, 2017
Richard Ward

ACKNOWLEDGEMENTS

EVERY PEBBLE THROWN in a pond makes a circle of ripples that flow outward in a never ending cycle of circles. Every human life makes an unending circle of ripples that flow outward in a never ending cycle of circles. We all become intertwined in the flow and ebb of the natural nature of ripples. No life is lived alone. Every stream of life flows and touches those with whom they wash against.

I am happy to have been touched by the circle of ripples of those who believe in my passion for our Stage 4 Breast Cancer women and their families.

They are a tribute to John Donne's beautiful poem:

> No man is an island,
> Entire of itself,
> Every man is a piece of the continent,
> A part of the main.
> If a clod be washed away by the sea,
> Europe is the less.
> As well as if a promontory were.
> As well as if a manor of thy friend's
> Or of thine own were:
> Any man's death diminishes me,
> Because I am involved in mankind,
> And therefore never send to know for whom the bell tolls;
> It tolls for thee.

I thank our 43 authors who told me they couldn't write. Read their words.

I thank our 3 editors, Julie Blamphin, Lauren Huffmaster, Stage 4 Breast Cancer, and Sarah Levinson, Stage 4 Breast Cancer, who have little vacant time in their occupied lives. I praise them for their dedication and fluency in polishing these written words.

I thank the children who wrote their small bits of love about their mothers. Imagine that!

I thank the husbands who stand between their dying wives and their families displaying silent strength outside while they writhe in pain inside.

I thank Danielle Joyner our graphic artist of extraordinary talent. She directed the *Anonymous Artistes* who helped to illustrate this book with her. Her sensitive touch and profound artistic gifts bring images and vibrancy to these stories.

"Those who say it can't be done, should get out of the way of those who are doing it."

62409409R00089

Made in the USA
Columbia, SC
02 July 2019